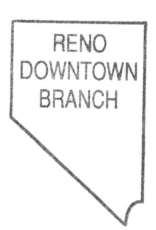

# Learning to Dance With the Dragonfly

# Learning to Dance With the Dragonfly

## Healing Lessons of Nature

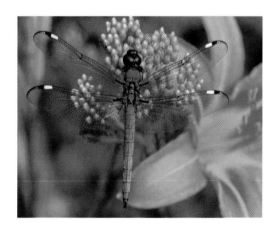

## Holly N. Fordyce

DANCING DRAGONFLY PRESS
*Carlisle, Massachusetts*

Although the author and publisher have made every effort to ensure the accuracy and completeness of information contained in this book, we assume no responsibility for errors, inaccuracies, omissions, or any inconsistency herein. Any slights of people, places, or organizations are unintentional.

First printing 2003

ISBN 0-9727013-4-6
LCCN 2002116586

**ATTENTION CORPORATIONS, UNIVERSITIES, COLLEGES, AND PROFESSIONAL ORGANIZATIONS:** Quantity discounts are available on bulk purchases of this book for educational, gift purposes, or as premiums for increasing magazine subscriptions or renewals. Special books or book excerpts can also be created to fit specific needs. For information, please contact Dancing Dragonfly Press, 867 Curve Street, Carlisle, MA 01741; ph. 978-369-8517.

With profound gratitude I dedicate *Learning to Dance With the Dragonfly* to creatures of the earth, sky and sea who touch my life and heal my spirit by reminding me I am connected to all that breathe here on this Earth our home.

## ACKNOWLEDGMENTS

With deep gratitude I want to thank all those dear readers with whom I shared the ragged first drafts of a book yet to sport a title through to its final version. Their unflagging support and friendship kept me afloat throughout the process of uncovering and discovery.

I'm indebted to poet Martha Dolben for sharing with me her insightful and keenly sensitive critical skills when fine-tuning both the prose and the poetry in this book. She provided me with an invaluable sounding board during our twice-monthly meetings when we shared and critiqued each other's writing.

My husband, Barry Ohs, deserves more hugs and kisses than he'll ever know for cheering me along every step of the way down the bog trail and for patiently listening to each piece as it was produced, then reading and rereading later versions. His persistent encouragement helped me stay passionate and focused.

# CONTENTS

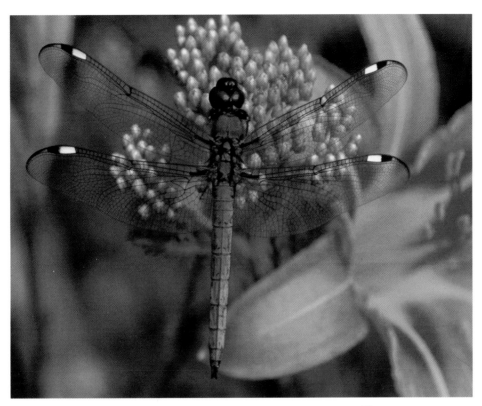

## Dancing With the Dragonfly

The dragonfly said *dance.*
She lit on my finger.
*Breathe the earth's blue air and dance*
*through brambles, eat blackberries*
*until your lips purple with wild sweet juices.*
*Sniff honeysuckle and apple blossoms.*
*Watch petals fall and remember them.*
Then up on cobwebbed wings
she hovered before me and whirled
across the ebony pond.

So I dance to the music of wild musicians,
to the songs of coyotes, thrushes and whales;
I sway in the wind with black-eyed Susans,
sniff milkweed, wild roses and mint.
I eat berries from thorny green brambles,
climb tangled arbors for grapes
and my lips turn purple and tingle.
I love what I love and dream
when I'm done
of dancing with a dragonfly
across an ebony pond.

# A Transformation Begins

On a perfect May afternoon in 1993, I telephoned the doctor for the results of a recent biopsy.

Her cheery greeting was quickly followed by a crisp clinical tone. "I'm sorry, the pathology report came back and it's not good." My body went limp, my heart stopped. The doctor offered to clear her busy schedule should my husband and I wish to speak to her in person that evening. I stopped listening. I could barely breathe. I had breast cancer.

Sun poured through an open window where a cardinal chipped at the feeder hanging nearby. I hung up the phone and plunged into a place of pure and thoughtless terror. Nothing was real—the cardinal, a splash of scarlet, flew away. My legs still held me up and I paced frantically from room to room, suffocating with fear and hearing my faraway voice crying, "Oh my God, oh my God" even before the tears came.

On this bright Tuesday afternoon when the light was so blue it hurt your eyes to look at it, I no longer felt comfortable in my own skin. My body had betrayed me and now felt alien and threatening. The tenuous sense of control I'd once known dropped off like an old coat. Suddenly in this season of beginnings, of giddy possibility, thoughts of death filled my mind with a noxious refrain. This magical month when I live in my garden and dig in the earth, loving its moist raw fragrance, when I plant seeds filled with surprise for the months to come, when I'm surrounded by birdsong wild as a symphony, became a backdrop to terror.

My husband rushed home from his work as soon as he heard my voice on the phone. With time to spare before our meeting with the doctor, we drifted out of the house and down the road to the cranberry bog. A small breeze lifted the still lacy leaves, Canada geese shepherded their families of tiny goslings through the black pond leaving little riffles of water in their wakes. Bobolinks called to one another across the meadow sending their liquid notes into the air. We didn't speak and I couldn't see for the tears clouding my eyes. The newly dressed trees, the lilting songs filling the moment felt distant and barely touched my senses.

Later in the afternoon sitting in the doctor's snowy office, I felt meek with fear as she told me my breast would have to be removed. In fifty-three years I'd never had surgery. While she assured me she would fashion a new breast better than the old one, I resisted an overpowering urge to vomit and demurred when asked to make an appointment for immediate surgery. We left her office, never to return.

The next day, clutching a packet of medical records, my husband drove me to Boston to meet another doctor. She pierced my despair with words of hope and was less eager to deface my body than the first doctor. I was a candidate for a partial mastectomy and radiation. I could do this.

In the following weeks I went on a frantic search for information about breast cancer and its treatment, both allopathic and alternative. More doctors, more tests and more decisions filled my days. One doctor supported my decision not to have surgery on my lymph nodes and forgo chemotherapy, while another ranted at me for going against protocol and refused to treat me. As the days passed and weeks went by my initial panic turned into blunted fear drumming in the background of each day as I focused on getting over the next hurdle. Often I woke up suddenly in the middle of the night, my breath stopped and my heart beating furiously. It really wasn't a dream. I really did have cancer.

In October, six months after my initial diagnosis, on the anniversary of mother's death, I had the last radiation treatment. It was over. I felt an enormous sense of relief. Now I could get on with living. Sleep came easier and I woke each morning, straightened the bed, plumped the pillows, watered the plants, fed my dog and put out seed for the birds before I went to work. But these comfortably mundane tasks became tinged with doom. Something was missing: I wasn't the same person and didn't know the one I'd become in such a short time.

When dressing, the indelible ink tattoos that ringed my deformed breast—tattoos pricked into my skin to guide the x-ray machine—reminded me of that ordeal. A third of its original size and flattened by scar tissue with a nipple collapsed on itself, never again to stand erect, my breast daily testified to my fragile mortality. Today I wear it as a badge of courage. The fear that once spread like hot molasses through my body has cooled and I no longer feel myself holding my breath and letting it out in a gushing sigh.

My vocabulary has spawned two pregnant words: "recurrence" fills me with dread and "survivor" conjures up hope. Recently I've learned that "cure" will not to be added to my lexicon. Where breast cancer is concerned, I must grasp the notion that I should accept living with a "chronic condition." This infuriates me. Whatever caused the cancer—and the possibilities are myriad—why, with all of our sophisticated medical technology, must we still cut it out, burn it and poison it? It rankles my spirit that prevention isn't a priority.

I've spent a long time finding ways to make life normal, to live with scarring, disfigurement and numbness in my breast, which once tingled with delicious sensations. But it's taken an even longer time to force myself to learn to live with uncertainty, the knowledge that a nasty cell may again invade my body and lurks even now, in some dark recess of my vulnerable self. My clock ticks just a bit faster than it used to. Breast cancer has had a profound impact on my life. It's changed me emotionally, physically and psychologically forever. The body I'd trusted and taken for granted betrayed me and yet, as the years pass, I know it's a good body. Encroaching age and disease may have brought recognition of life's uncertainty and poured fuel on my angst about mortality, but here I am "with miles to go before I sleep."

While healing began with medical treatment and continued with alternative medicines, it's taken other forms as well. At first I started a journal into which I poured all my anger, hurt and fear. I've been filled with rage, rage at the unfairness of what's happened to me, rage at losing the last remnant of innocence that kept me a safe distance from death. I was afraid the cancer would return, afraid I'd be further disfigured, suffer unpalliated pain and worst of all, I'd lose my self entirely to fear. My soul shook. I was angry with others who went on with their lives leaving me behind to wrestle with my new demons. I was afraid to speak of my fears to those I loved the most and on whom I so depended. It seemed to me they couldn't entertain the idea of recurrence and didn't want to fear for me. While I needed to respect their feelings, I needed so badly to have witnesses who could tolerate me as I struggled to find a new way to be. I wanted to bare my disfigured breast without shame.

While family relationships weighed heavily on my spirit for several years, my friendships were a tonic. I worried sadness would depress my immune system and invite the cancer to return. I worried for myself and for those I loved who were in their own pain-filled worlds as I typed page after page of muttering and grumbling and whimpering into my computer. Months turned into years of readjustment. I'm a slow learner. I spent a lot of energy taking care of my body with diet, herbs, vitamins, exercise and the most precious support of friends who could be with me. Bouts of therapy helped me make some sense of what was happening to me, but after a few years, I was still adrift. One day I read over the pages I'd written and felt worse than ever. I was terribly stuck and needed a place to tuck away the betrayal and anger that distorted my life. I desperately needed to find what was missing. I needed a new focus. First, I looked to see who was right outside my window. The cardinals had returned and now there were four pairs flashing their wings in the sunlight. I bought a lovely leather-bound notebook and began to write in longhand. Wielding a silver pen, I could feel words slide across a clean white page. It made me feel more connected to the words that tumbled out of my head and lay in a heap on the page. I could walk on my two feet, take up my camera to stalk bees and dragonflies and wait for a wildflower to stop nodding in the breeze so it could be captured on film. Most important, I was nurturing and being nurtured by good friendships.

I wrote about my nature observations during daily walks with my golden retriever, Rosie. Taking a cue from Henry Thoreau who wrote in his journal, on November 16, 1850, "My journal should be the record of my love. I would write in it only of the things I love, my affection for any aspect of the world, what I love to think of…," I too would write of what I loved. The pages of the journal brimmed with thoughts and observations and quotes and poems that touched me.

One book filled then another and I began to notice something profound happening to me. Moments of clarity snuck up on me and little by little laughter returned. I clung to the hope that with careful nurturing my immune system might actually outsmart a recurrence of cancer. Writing propelled me on a quest that had eluded me for years—the search for my spirit. I began to understand that my life did not have to be driven by being happy or unhappy, bored or filled to the brim, or even consumed with anxiety. I was not a billboard for breast cancer; there were many facets of me other than disease and while I could no longer count on tomorrow, I would not wait for the future before living the way I wanted to live. I could gather moments and practice exquisite awareness while life dared me to live more on its edge. Moved to feel gratitude for being alive, I was compelled to talk to the geese and greet the great blue heron, even speak to dragonflies as they went about their business down at the cranberry bog. When these creatures tolerated my presence, even stopped to take notice, I felt I had been given something special. Walking closely with a friend, sharing our selves and breathing the season's air for yet another miraculous year was a gift I had not recognized as such until now.

Capturing what presented itself to me through the lens of my spirit as well as that of my camera brought me into the moment. Paying attention to what was before me, learning to really see brought me out of my shadow into moments where I felt truly joyful. I was able to hold fear at bay for days, even months. What is written here is a journal-memoir of thoughts, feelings and memories that blossomed during a year walking into nature where I could safely delve into deep places of my heart to find where its spirit lies.

# January

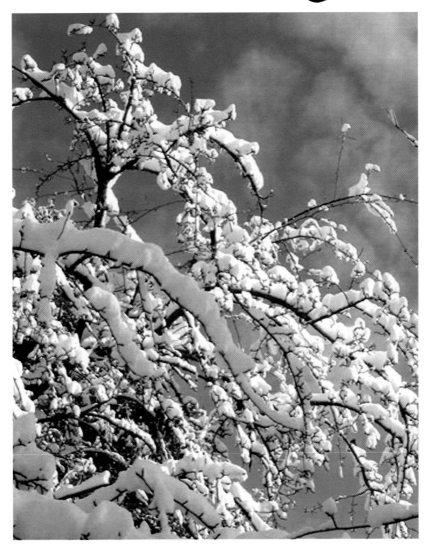

"In the midst of winter I discovered in me an invincible summer."

*Albert Camus*

# A Place in the Heart

"What would the world be, once bereft
Of wet and of wildness? Let them be left
O let them be left, wildness and wet;
Long live the weeds and the wilderness yet."
*Gerard Manley Hopkins*

Letting the screen door slam behind us, Rosie and I head for the cranberry bog. A quarter of a mile down a country road from my house is a large parcel of land occupying part of the northwest border of Carlisle, a small village west of Boston. The bog is an old one and using rather haphazard farming techniques has yielded a respectable harvest of deep red cranberries early in November for many years. Recently the town has acquired the bog and its surrounding woodland and turned it into conservation land except for the cranberry meadows, which are leased to a local farmer.

Rounding the curve in the road Rosie and I come upon the imposing and venerable bog-house wrapped in weathered shingles and overlooking the cranberry meadows whose broad, flat acreage comprises a unique blend of habitats. Marshes, two ponds and a forest border the meadows. Where these habitats merge, large and diverse numbers of creatures come to find food, to mate and raise their young. The trail Rosie and I daily walk winds around cranberry meadows, fallow fields, alongside ponds and into the woods if we're up for a longer walk.

Attracted to the bog and its environs are animals who make their homes in the mud in the bottom of the ponds or in the tangle of weeds growing along their banks or among the cat-o'-nine-tails springing out of their swampy edges; others make nests in hummocks of grass or inside the low shrubs that grow in the fallow meadows. Many creatures live in the branches of maple, oak and pine trees that line the forest's edge. Deeper in the forest, hawks, crows and squirrels build huge nests high in tops of white pines. Finally, lizards and small rodents burrow into the sandy shoulders of the trails or dig into the thick leaf litter to make their homes.

Separated from smaller, fallow meadows by dirt causeways, the productive cranberry field stretches its velvet carpet of ground-hugging plants over several acres, which turn light green in the spring and deepen in color until in the fall, the meadow becomes wine red. Carved into the nap of the carpet is a network of small, interconnected irrigation ditches, which are fed by a broad central ditch several yards wide. This large wing of water runs south to north and is in turn, filled with the overflow of the southern and largest of two ponds bordering the bog. Here the water is deep and clear. Minnows can be seen darting in and out of the waving bottom grasses. Families of mallards glide up and down its length and clutches of Canada geese graze along its banks. The working meadow is flooded or drained depending on the cranberry plants' need for water or protection from killing frosts. When the wooden dam that holds back the pond is lifted, water gushes through a large silver duct into the big ditch, then runs more slowly into the smaller ones until the meadow is flooded. Most of the time these little ditches lie like ribbons of still, shallow water gleaming in the sun with an oily skim of rainbow-colored residue. I think it's either an artifact of the acid soil type or, God forbid, the result of something worse and toxic.

Trotting ahead of me with her tail high as a flag, Rosie startles a great blue heron fishing for frogs in the small ditch running the length of the dike road, which separates the south pond from the meadow. The bird lurches into the air and slowly flaps off to land at the edge of another ditch. We continue on, each of us focused on our own interests. No odor escapes Rosie's nose and I too try not to let anything escape any of my five senses. We've now reached the northern wooded border of the bog meadow and arrive at the upper pond. Its swampy edges are filled with reeds, waterlogged stumps and fallen tree limbs where painted turtles string themselves in a necklace of large, glossy beads to warm themselves in the sun. Herons are particularly fond of fishing here in the quiet shallows camouflaged by clumps of tall cat-o'-nine-tails. Bunches of purple loosestrife grow in an ever-thickening mass around the perimeter of this once large pond. Not far from its shore, mats of water lily pads clot the open water; their creamy flowers have wangled their way through the murky water into the light. Each year this pond shrinks a little more as plants crowd into the water and decaying matter consumes precious oxygen. While populations of larger fish decline, the encroaching vegetation with its thicket of weeds is a haven for frogs, small fry, beaver, herons, nesting geese, ducks and all kinds of songbirds.

I've lived by the cranberry bog for many years and even in its wilder days, it produced a good crop of berries and supported a large and diverse population of wildlife as well. Some years, great flotillas of Canada geese floated on both ponds and bright yellow hatchlings paddled close to their mothers. Come June yellow-hatted bobolinks sang their silvery notes from the tops of bushes growing in the fallow meadows. Today as Rosie and I make our way around these patches thick with grasses and abundant wildflowers, I listen with joy tinged with sadness to the songs of diminishing flocks of sparrows: Chipping sparrows, song sparrows, white-throated sparrows and swamp sparrows hurry to raise and fledge young before the farmer's mowing blade slices their protective shelters to the ground. Only one bobolink sings on the wing. Only at the wood's edge do numbers of goldfinch, kingfishers and warblers dart in and out of the trees and hide in the under-story thickets to sing their love songs.

In the clean sky above us, a red-tailed hawk glides in wide circles over the meadows scanning the fields below, biding its time until it spots a small movement in the grass below and plunges out of the sky to grab a hapless mouse skittering for home. Several species of hawks, American kestrels and turkey vultures circle the bog at various times of the year. Some are residents and others pass through the neighborhood on their way south in the fall or north to cooler climes in spring.

Attracted to the wetlands in early spring, flocks of exuberant redwing blackbirds flash their scarlet wing patches and sway from the tips of cat-o'-nine-tails to call out for mates. Red foxes skulk about at twilight looking for rabbits that have become scarcer as the fox population has increased. I imagine the tide will turn and foxes will search for more abundant feeding grounds. Either way I miss the rabbits and I'll miss the lovely rusty, bushy-tailed foxes trotting across these fields. At sunset white-tailed deer join other evening creatures and venture out of the woods to drink from the ponds and graze the banks of the ditches. Once in a while when I walk at dusk, I'm startled by what sounds like a gunshot as I approach the upper pond. A beaver smacks his tail on the water to warn others of my intrusion.

Late spring on into fall huge, homely snapping turtles, small painted turtles, ribbon snakes and water snakes slide just beneath the skin of the pond's surface. Often I see turtles drag themselves out of the water onto the sandy shoulders of the trails to lay their eggs. Of the scores of insects that buzz and hover over the bog, most notable are the dragonflies and damselflies that have successfully kept a potentially prolific mosquito population under control, especially since pesticide spraying was banned in our town. Honey bees, beetles and all kinds of butterflies feed on the wildflowers growing at the edges of the ditches, in the fallow meadows and along the banks of the ponds.

Now the local farmer, to whom the cranberry bog has been leased, is making a determined effort to rehabilitate the fallow cranberry patches and farm the still productive meadow so as to produce a profitable harvest. Until recently, both herbicides and pesticides have been used to control weeds and insect pests during the summer months. There have been times when I've had to forgo my daily walk around the bog trails because the odor of chemicals was so strong coming off the field. Even more disturbing for me was learning of the high incidence of breast cancer occurring on Cape Cod where there are numerous cranberry farms. While I choose not to walk the bog trails when chemicals are in use, and I can afford not to drink my cold well water any longer for fear that the ground water may be contaminated, I worry about the creatures who have no choice—creatures whose livelihoods depend on uncontaminated water and the growth of plants and shrubs that provide food and shelter. I worry that their habitats are not only being poisoned, but are being destroyed by the mowing blade. Certainly this spring I've noticed even fewer birds nesting in and around the bog. Only two Canada goose families produced small clutches of goslings. The rafts of cackling geese are gone. Just as noticeably absent are the butterflies. The ubiquitous fritillaries, who only last year, massed around dandelion blossoms in search of nectar are fewer in number.

As Rosie and I round the meadows and head toward home, I can only imagine how many other species have been harmed or affected in some way by the rehabilitation of the cranberry farm. So, just as damaging as use of chemicals, is the reclamation of the small, forgotten meadows now razored clean, which last year were covered with thick shrubs, hummocks of grass and an abundance of wildflowers; thistle, a favorite of goldfinches, mullein and milkweed, joe-pie weed, maple and oak saplings have all been mowed down. This once extraordinarily unique home for wild creatures and flora has fast become less hospitable as its ecosystem is managed and manipulated by human intervention.

In his book, *In Search of Nature*, Edward O. Wilson writes, "The human species is, in a word, an environmental hazard…" (p. 186). "When we debase the global environment and extinguish the variety of life, we are dismantling a support system that is too complex to understand, let alone replace, in the foreseeable future" (p. 190). The main cause of increasing mass extinctions of wild creatures, he says, is because of "the destruction of natural habitat….Close behind, is the introduction of…exotic organisms (such as purple loosestrife) that outbreed and extirpate native species" (p. 194). "Even a small loss in area," Wilson says, "reduces the number of species. The relation is such that when the area of habitat is cut to one-tenth of its original cover, the number of species eventually drops by roughly one-half" (p. 195). "Extinction is now proceeding thousands of times faster than the production of new species….Humanity is now destroying most of the habitats where evolution can occur" (p.196).

Rosie and I head home and I think how twenty-five years ago when I first moved here, the cranberry bog was a wild place, a place I took for granted as I hiked its trails, unaware then of the treasures it offered up to anyone who took time to look. I used to shake the grape vines and grapes would tumble into my shopping bag. In July I filled a bucket with blueberries. And the bog was a place to exercise when the spirit moved me. While the blueberry shrubs have been cut down, the grape vines still climb to the sun, but these days they produce less fruit.

I suspect when there's less demand for a cash crop, less rigorous farming methods will end up being more economical and once again the bog will comfortably support both a productive cranberry business and the creatures that once made it their home. The edge habitat, once unique and prolific, will again become hospitable to diverse populations of wildlife and plants.

As we turn into our driveway, Gus, our other golden retriever, trots up to greet us. Barry, my husband and companion of twenty years, pokes his head out of his workshop at the back of the garage. These two accompany Rosie and me on weekend walks around the bog. Sometimes we venture further afield into other conservation areas. Barry is learning to tolerate my wish to practice walking in silence and like mine, his sensory experiences have sharpened over the months we've traversed the bog trails with more attention.

Gus acts as Rosie's elderly uncle, who graciously tolerates her exuberance and childish provocations and whose step has been considerably lightened by Rosie's demand for a playmate. Rosie rushes up to Gus, sniffs him and finding nothing of interest, trots over to Barry to have her ears scratched. I will be forever indebted to Barry, who presented me with this golden puppy three years ago, a creature whose boundless joy infects me daily. Rosie kisses noses and in return likes her ears and the soft place between her eyes kissed. She has a way of gazing at me until I must, and often do, guess what it is she desires, which is most often food, a chance to walk or just to be close to me.

I leave the dogs outside to wrestle on the grass and go into the house where two Himalayan cats sit like statues in the doorway. Patches greets me with a long, plaintive "meow." Hazel merely stares at me with her blue marble eyes. I ask them to let me by and one by one they rise to follow me into the porch where I sit down to take off my boots. Patches levitates onto my lap. She's a special cat with a smooshed-in, patchy face dominated by sapphire eyes, which command me to make eye contact when she speaks. She talks a great deal about love, pouring out endless purrs and soft cat noises to communicate her desire to huddle close and be stroked. She returns the favor with finger-licking kisses. Patches' slight frame appears deceptively large dressed in its cloud of silky, tawny fur that fluffs up and down like petticoats when she trots from room to room. Rosie yearns to make friends with Patches, but Patches is cautious, unwilling to be the object of a chase, yet happy to snuggle when Rosie is comatose. Hazel stays aloof from most of the family. Once a day she asks me to scratch behind her ears, then she disappears into a safe corner to sleep the hours away. She dislikes Rosie intensely and barely tolerates Gus. Now and again she warms up to Patches, but mostly she's our mysterious, dark recluse who when she purrs with pleasure, does so with such force, she chokes.

I count as residents all the creatures who live just outside my window, within my walls or in the dark unseen corners of my house. These include red and gray squirrels, the occasional family of raccoons who consider our chimney a suitable place to raise a family, the mice who scrabble and scratch within my walls all night long and the skunk who sneaks around at night perfuming the shrubs under my window while searching for birdseed. White-tailed deer often wander through the yard, sometimes stopping to nibble at apples I've tossed out for them in the winter. And once a black bear made midnight raids on our bird feeders and provided us with a week of entertainment. Then there are the myriad birds who come year-round to dine at the feeding stations surrounding the house. In warmer months, butterflies, dragonflies, mosquitoes and ants beguile and pester us. June bugs thrash against the screened windows and soft-winged moths cloud around the outside light. Crickets sing in the corners of the porch and night frogs offer lullabies until I'm wrapped in a soothing concert. This is my neighborhood, my home, and these are my family.

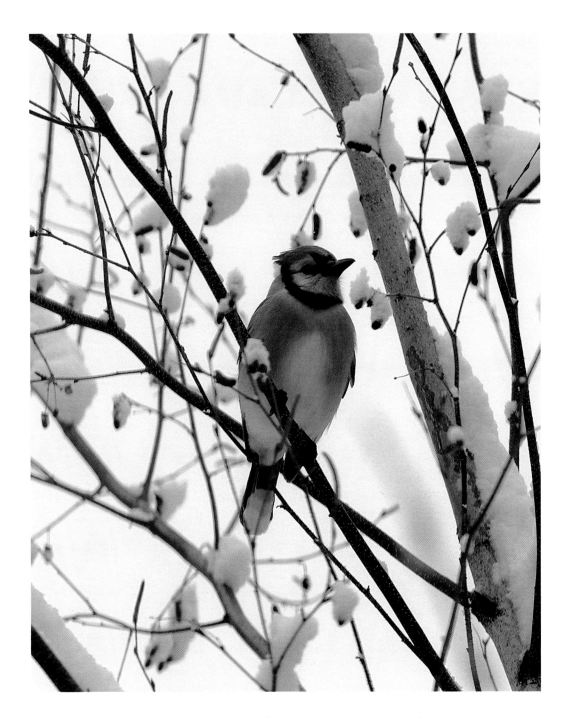

"In the presence of nature a wild delight runs through the person, in spite of real sorrows."

~ *Ralph Waldo Emerson*

# January Journal

### January 1

I want to learn to walk like Rosie does. No matter how many times we've walked the same bog trails, Rosie thinks we're on an adventure to an exotic place; every walk is filled with new delights and curiosities. If I think to pay attention as she does, I too can be transported by the same old vista seen in different lights with different eyes. So often my mind is rummaging through a jumble of thoughts that have nothing to do with where I am. When this happens, I'm reminded of Henry David Thoreau, who wrote in Walden, "I am alarmed when it happens that I have walked a mile into the woods bodily, without getting there in spirit." I'm working hard to keep my attention focused on my feet at least—putting one in front of the other, listening to the sound of each footfall on grass or leaves or gravel or snow. Perhaps I must hone my senses, feet first. My body walks for exercise and the effort of focusing exercises my mind.

Just as I turn out my lamp to go to sleep, I'm startled by a coyote's howl. They are skulking around the house again and punctuate the darkness with their eerie yips. I clutch Rosie close to me. Funny, how these wild creatures soon become undaunted by our proximity. I think coyotes may be as opportunistic as raccoons, who have dined on our cooped-up-chickens, raided our garbage cans and have been quite content to live off our leavings. Coyotes will even eat a pet cat.

### January 2

Today the fifty-degree temperature tempts me with the promise of spring. The air is soft and breezeless. Puddles collect in depressions in the ice-bound bog pond until the surface glistens. The sun, just visible behind a tattered quilt of retreating clouds, paints them scarlet and lavender as Rosie and I take a late afternoon walk through the mysterious, thick mist hovering over the flooded cranberry meadow where warm air has collided with the frozen land. The white goose and her adopted family of five Canada geese are poking at the melting ice looking for a stray cranberry. I'm sure it's the same little goose I saw last October.

I've discovered this bird is an immature snow goose who's more slender than her Canadian cousins; her white feathers are a bit on the grayish side and she has a black beak and dark legs. I wonder if the snow goose lost her family during the migration last fall. She's fortunate to have been welcomed into this resident group. Suddenly the six geese take off for the pond where they come in for a long sliding touch down on the watery ice. It looks like fun.

## January 6

Above me the oaks and maple trees throw a net of delicate black lace across the sky. Every twig is loaded with buds, more abundant than I remember in other years. Our capricious weather has coaxed a young maple sapling's buds to thrust tiny green leaves into the now bitter air. In the iced-in-cove where the reeds still stand in thick dry bunches, a great blue heron is on a futile search for something to eat.

## January 25

A spate of bitter cold has bought with it days and nights of sharp wind and a few inches of snow. When there's a lull in the biting wind, Rosie and I make our way to the bog. The path along the meadow is strewn with frozen honeybees lured out of their hives by the warming sun. I want to ask the bee man, who tends several hives set along the perimeter of the cranberry meadow, why his bees were so foolish as to venture out into the cold to die. I ponder this until my thoughts are interrupted by the strident voices of a pair of crows wheeling over the meadows fighting the thickening wind blowing in from the northwest. The heron is gone and so are the geese.

The snow makes everything look lovely. Most of my clients canceled their appointments, not wanting to drive in this weather, so I sit at my window watching birds crowd around the feeding stations. I've noticed how different species of birds take turns coming to the feeders and how the same birds frequent the same feeders. Earliest at the suet cakes hung outside the porch windows is a pair of brown Carolina wrens, tiny and round who sing all winter long when other birds simply call to one another. Then come the nuthatches and a downy woodpecker. The little birds tend to feed first before the larger ones bully them away.

A bevy of drab house sparrows clings to the long seed feeders gorging on sunflower kernels. They scatter in a sudden flurry of wings when a blue jay plunges out of the spruce across the driveway to grab a seed. Slate-colored juncos and a pair of gentle mourning doves scratch in the snow looking for spilled seed. At the side of the house four pairs of cardinals dominate the feeding trays. Now they loiter in the shelter of a large hemlock before descending to scatter the other birds away. A scarlet male poses on a deep green and snow-dusted branch while his more modestly clad mate has her turn at the feeding station. A flock of goldfinches dressed in olive winter attire gathers around several thistle-seed feeders hanging outside another window where I can watch them.

Recently, I've bought a long telephoto lens for my camera. I have set the camera on a tripod for stability and placed the apparatus at the open window in the porch door and wait. If I'm quiet and hide behind the curtain covering the door, I'm able to capture a portrait of a cardinal or a chickadee or a woodpecker. This stalking game is exciting, but it's not easy to photograph chickadees and titmice, which are quick and fidgety as they dash in for a seed and zip away before I've even focused my lens. It's going to take some practice and infinitely more patience than I'm used to having. I'm determined to get the hang of it. My fingers are stiff from holding the icy barrel of the lens and my back aches from holding myself immobile. Then joy comes when, through the lens, I look a cardinal in the eye and snap his photograph without disturbing his lunch.

## January 30

Once again it's lovely and warm. The thermometer has risen from an icy fifteen degrees to a temperate forty-five, although more snow is predicted for tomorrow. I feel restless and don't know quite why. It's been a quiet month, a good one, a month free of worries, yet for some reason sleep has become elusive lately and I wake at odd hours of the night. Maybe I've begun an inward journey again. Sometimes when I embark on these thinking trips without prior warning, I slip into a mindfulness I hadn't expected and which I look forward to. Being alone much of this month with Barry away some of the time and me not walking as frequently as I wished may also account for my moodiness.

# Water

I come from water, once
a sea-nymph rocking
in my mother's amniotic pool.
My blood streams
out in tiny capillary fingers
like a river delta, it pours into a tangle
of veins and arteries to fill my heart.
Cells bathed in water rush in and out
from every pore, every opening and menstrual bloods
surge like moon tides.
Twice my womb held a fragile gift in a lagoon
bound by its permeable membrane and twice my breasts
were swelled with milk and suckled by persistent mouths.
Now ocean tears spatter my cheek with streaks of white.
Parched and tired, I quench my thirst from Earth's springs,
lick raindrops, swallow snowflakes and drink
and drink and drink.

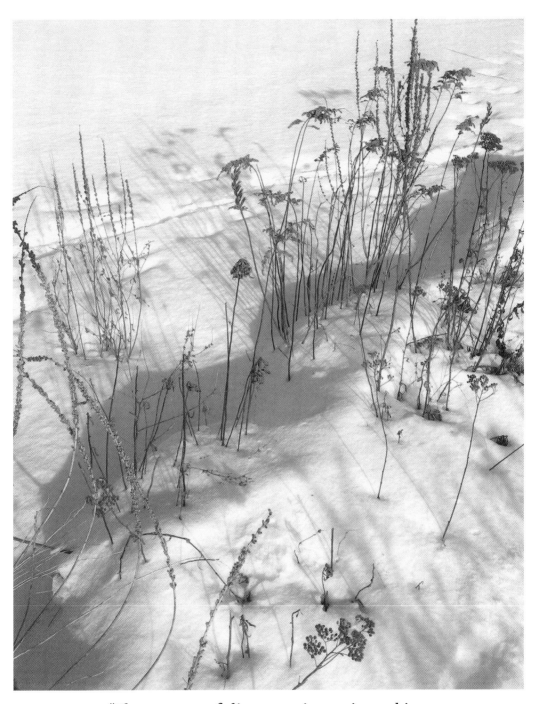

"The voyage of discovery is not in seeking
new landscapes but in having new eyes."

*Marcel Proust*

# The Fairy Clock

I dream of flying. I glide up and over trees so close I can touch their topmost leaves with the tips of my toes. I soar over a patchwork of green fields, meadows and along a wide, slow river. I'm not afraid of falling because when I tire, I float down and land in the water like a Canada goose with my feet straight out before me and slide across the surface until I step out of the river onto a grassy bank. Then all of a sudden, I'm awake. I want to fly again.

This dream began years ago when I was very young and my mother told me the story of the fairy clock sitting on a narrow mantel over a small fireplace in her bedroom. Flanking the little clock was a pair of candelabra hung with crystal prisms. When the sun found them and a breeze snuck in through the summer window they tinkled and sent sparkling rainbows along the walls and across the ceiling.

The fairy clock was no more than five inches high. Its thick crystal sides were framed in delicately filigreed brass. I could look inside the clock and see its coiled springs and watch toothed wheels go around and around. Tic-toc, tic-toc, tic-toc—it ticked off the seconds until on the hour the clock sang a gentle chime to mark the time and again, on the half hour. With a special brass key, my mother wound the fairy clock once a week. To do this she opened a glass door at the back of the clock. I was warned never to touch the key and never, ever the clock.

Back then my mother was between husbands so my little sister and I often rose early in the morning and tapped on our mother's bedroom door until she drowsily called us in. We ran pell-mell into the room and leaped onto her enormous bed—usually me first, since I was the fastest and the oldest. Vying loudly for the place closest to our mother, we forgot she had two sides, one for each of us to snuggle against. Thankfully, my mother loved to cuddle. I remember her warm and sleepy smell early in the morning. She'd giggle as my sister and I mimicked her long stretching yawns before settling under the covers for a story. Now and again she read fairy tales from a book, but the best stories she made up, stories about rabbits and little people who lived in the woods across the field from our house.

One day my sister took sick and had to stay in bed. On this morning I had my mother all to myself. Wrapped in her warm covers and lying as close to her as I could get, I begged for a story.

"I'll tell you about the fairy clock if you promise not to wiggle." The fairy clock was a very old and delicate French traveling clock that belonged to a great lady who took it with her when she journeyed around the world.

"Remember, Holly, you must never touch it. If you do," said my mother, "you'll upset the little people who live inside and they won't dance to the chimes."

"What little people?" I asked incredulously.

"The fairies, of course!" she replied. "They live inside among the wheels and when the clock chimes you can hear tiny voices sing. You can even hear the patter of their little feet dancing. But you have to be quiet as a mouse, not a peep." I climbed out of her warm bed and stood close to the fairy clock on the mantel. Suddenly, the chime rang in my ear.

"Mummy, I don't hear anything!"

My mother laughed with delight. "Maybe you're not being quiet enough."

From that day on, I never thought of the little brass clock as a mere timepiece. It was magic. It housed the fairies of my mother's imagination, little people who danced and sang around their queen under the umbrella of a giant mushroom.

Fairies lived in the woods too. Sometimes my mother and I pretended we were very small with dragonfly wings sprouting from our backs. We'd talk to each other in squeaky voices and she was always the queen.

When I'm lonely or sad, I imagine myself in a pine forest curled up in a warm blanket of velvet green moss beneath the shadow of a tall brown toadstool, the kind with pale fluted underskirts. I drift off to sleep listening to chickadees "dee-deeing" and warblers warbling and the chatter of little winged creatures humming around my head wondering who I am. I've always wanted to fly through the woods up over the treetops, high above fields and meadows, to sail like a bird.

The fairy clock now sits on my desk in my bedroom. I still listen for the magical little voices when it chimes. I still dream of flying.

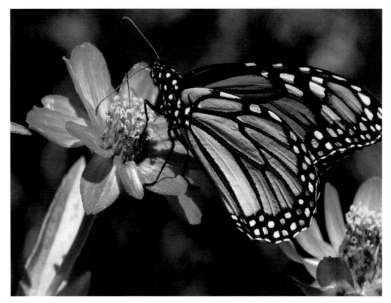

## Flight

She held the jar to the window.
Inside, bound with silken threads
its shell thin as glass,
a folded butterfly
clutched a sprig of milkweed.

"Look!" she cried.
The skin split, fell away and monarch wings
unfurled and fanned the air.
Out in the garden,
my mother uncapped the jar.

How she knew, I'll never know
And one day she was gone;
her diaries incinerated, rose
page by seventy years of pages
of hunger and secrets.

Briefly she hovered
on unfamiliar wings
awaiting the small wind
that lifted her away.

22

# February

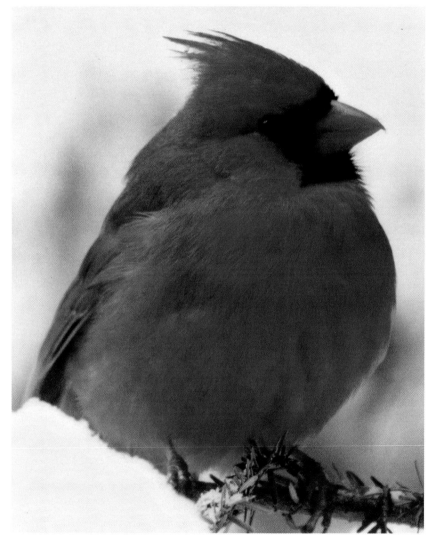

"Nature is the nature of all things that are; things that are have a union with all things from the beginning."

ᴄ *Marcus Aurelius*

# February Journal

### February 6

I've been practicing with my large telephoto lens and am privy to an intimate view of my subject. It's like spying. I'm quite certain I see expressions on some bird faces. Chickadees, for instance, look playfully intent and curious, and sometimes startled.

Lately I've been thinking about my favorite of the small birds, the black-capped chickadee, paying particular attention to its language. I always know when fall is coming even before leaves begin to change color because chickadees announce the season with "chick-a-dee-dee-dee" as they signal to one another it's time to gather in flocks for the cold months ahead. In late winter, when male chickadees break away from their flocks to begin marking their breeding territories, they sing, "fee-bee." Two clear notes fill the woods around my house and announce spring is near. These calls are the chickadee's most notable vocalizations, but they can also be heard scolding or even whispering softly to one another when feeding.

The chickadee's body language is charming. I've seen a feisty male open his sharp little beak, crouch low like a boxer and stick his head out to frighten another bird away. A courting female shivers her wings to catch the attention of a nearby male and when she dances like this, he will come so close to her they touch beaks as if kissing. Sometimes he brings her a gift of food.

By mid-spring mated pairs of chickadees have finished building their nests and lay their clutch of eggs. I've never found a nest, perhaps because these smart birds remove all signs of their nest building and I've never seen a baby chickadee either. Once their young have fledged, chickadees hang out with tufted titmice and other small birds like nuthatches and downy woodpeckers and return to my feeders to consume pounds of sunflower seed and suet.

### February 13

Rosie nudges me for her breakfast. I stretch and yawn, not wanting to rise quite yet, but my nose is wet from insistent licking and now Patches has been disturbed. I have no recourse but to heave myself out of bed. Stretching legs stiff with morning arthritis, I limp into the kitchen and put a scoop of kibble in Rosie's bowl and offer it to her after a sit-down and a nose kiss. Once she's finished, I let her outdoors and quickly crawl back under the warm covers where Patches waits to settle again on my pillow to purr in my ear. Overhead I hear a familiar honking. A flock of geese wings across the sky window, their white underbellies glistening in the sun.

Just as I pick up my book, Rosie makes it clear she's ready to come in. Her pitiful whine and yips demand immediate entry. When this fails, she jumps up to peer at me through the door window looking like a funny cartoon character with two paws, a nose and a pair of imploring eyes visible. I let her in and she hops up on the bed and stretches out beside me and Patches.

Now and again they wake from their naps to sniff or lick one another before turning their wet attention to me. I'm pinned down by these creatures and feel too claustrophobic to doze off myself or even to read comfortably, but I dare not budge lest I disturb this moment of heaven I share with Rosie and Patches. I can't imagine my life without them in it.

Our peaceful nap is over when Barry comes to let Gus out. With a mug of coffee in hand, he settles down in his chair to read. By now it's mid-morning and the porch is glowing with light. A hyacinth, blue as a sapphire, blooms by the window. On the table, a bouquet of white lilies, orange dust dropping onto their newly opened petals, sends a waft of fragrance to mingle with the intoxicating scent of the hyacinth. If I look carefully enough, I see minute iridescences in the petals of pink and blue and lavender primroses growing in pots that line the windowsills.

I get to work on a small quilt for my first grandbaby, who is expected in April. I congratulate myself on its straight seams and matching corners. Years ago my quilts were sewn on an antique treadle machine and accurate measuring was neglected in favor of speed and an impatient desire to see the final result. I've decided to sew this gift by hand and with each stitch I imagine what it will be like to be a grandmother and knowing her gender (already determined by ultrasound) I wonder what she'll be like. I dream of her, how much I want to show her, to teach her about birds, flowers and nature—all the miracles of nature that captivated my mother and now bewitch me again.

When my children were small, I was less patient and too preoccupied with responsibility to nurture my passion for nature and her creatures. My curiosity and drive to know things were distracted and overwhelmed by events, which shocked my naive fifties' sensibilities into the turbulent sixties and seventies. Women's liberation, civil rights and the Vietnam War hotly competed in my mind with new environmental concerns after I'd read *Silent Spring*. I became an opinionated inactivist who read and studied and thought about all that was happening around me until I became just knowledgeable enough to develop large convictions about large and relevant issues and became loudly vocal about all of them. But that was all. There were so many causes, I ended up stewing in my own shame for not having the courage to march for even one of them. My children, wrapped in their own growing needs and unaware of their mother's stunted passions, were helplessly perplexed as their worlds collapsed when I stumbled into divorce and when hurtled toward a fearsome unknown, convinced this would pry me out of a deepening depression. It didn't.

Overwhelmed by these memories, suddenly I'm in one of those moods where I have to move furniture, rearrange things, clean up and clear out. I vacuum dirt and debris behind and under places that haven't been cleaned in months. Every now and again, ceasing this frenetic motion I stand by the camera aimed at the viburnum twigs and wait for a bird willing to pose for me. Then it's back to pushing and shoving, pulling and throwing out until I'm sweating with the effort in spite of the open window. Early afternoon sun floods into the porch and gives the room a luminous quality. I'm happy, really happy at this moment. The changes I've made are satisfying, the nooks and crannies are clean and all that was torn apart has been rearranged in a pleasing order. Still in my nightgown, now gray, I go to change into my jeans.

Barry comes in from his workshop at the back of the garage carrying a treasure box he's made for me. It's made of cherry wood and glows with polish. Gathering old and special letters, seashells, pebbles collected from my travels in Africa, feathers and, journals, colored pencils and an old Bible belonging to my grandfather, I fill the box. In the midst of collecting my treasures, I've come across a dust-covered oriole's nest found last summer by the roadside, which I pin to the wall in the porch. Blowing the dust off the nest, I arrange my collection of bird feathers in and around the nest cavity until the nest sprouts an odd, but spectacular bouquet of feathers dropped by blue jays, cardinals, sparrows, hawks, crows, gulls and a special feather from a Kenyan guinea fowl. In the nest cavity I place a blue and broken robin's eggshell.

After a late afternoon walk and a cup of tea, the day comes to an end. Darkness envelops the porch, the birds have found their shelters, supper is made and we dine by candlelight. A wonderful feeling of accomplishment fills me. It's been a good day.

## ~ *February 18*

Starlings have discovered the feeding station outside the porch. They are a scrappy, noisy bunch who fight with each other constantly. Except for their iridescent, blue-black feathers, funny faces and their penchant for flying in formation with more precision than the famous Thunderbirds, starlings are homely birds.

The trails around the bog have become treacherously slippery. A day of rain and a dusting of snow have prevented us from walking these past couple of days.

Tired of being cooped up Rosie nudges me, carries my boots around in her mouth until I agree to a walk . Showers of sunlight sparkle across the black pond where a light wind riffles the surface—the same wind that chased the clouds off this morning. Arrows of light fall between the pines and across the woods trail. We bushwhack through a thicket to a place where the bog swamp curves around the forest and an abandoned beaver hut hugs the shore. I've chosen this spot for a day of solitude in the spring.

Huddled with Rosie on the old rag rug I've brought, I lean against the trunk of a pine and she lies warm against my legs. Behind us a tangle of scrub makes us almost invisible. It's cold. Rosie's ears twitch to hear the small sounds carried on the wind inaudible to me. Two pairs of Canada geese poke around in the frozen reeds a few yards away. All of a sudden Rosie sits up and sniffs the air. I tell her to keep quiet—we don't want our special place to be found out. Twigs snap and I turn just in time to see a family of white-tailed deer trotting over the rise behind our hideaway. We're downwind of them so the deer are unaware of our presence. Rosie holds her tongue until they disappear. The wind picks up and so do I. A bowl full of gold-tinged clouds fills the pond and a red-tailed hawk sails high above the cranberry meadow calling "keer-keer." The chickadees who'd been bouncing along the trail with us singing their spring "fee-bee" song have gone silent and disappear into the shrubbery.

## ⟿ *February 22*

Walking across the dike beside the pond I hear the wing-song of a solitary Canada goose. The wind whooshes through her wings with each beat as she circles around and around the meadow honking mournfully. Not finding whatever or whoever she was looking for, the goose disappears over the tops of the pines. Because Canada geese pair for life, I feel terrible when I see a single goose like this one.

This week the wailing of chainsaws and the awful breaking of trees crashing to the ground herald the development of the woodlands behind my house. I'm furious at the intrusion of a crowd of ostentatious homes, which will invade our rural neighborhood, but most of all I'm angry at the destruction of forest habitat. Every time the saw ceases whining, a majestic tree cries out and plunges to the ground. It breaks my heart. Chopping down trees, even pruning shrubs, is always difficult for me, but this daily cracking and booming is too much. I slide a birdsong CD into the player and turn up the volume to drown out the sound.

It's hard to believe pastoral Carlisle is following the example of so many other towns whose fields and woodlands have sprouted mansions so fast it makes one's head spin. These arks rise out of denuded woodlands or in bare fields, each with its man-made hills built over a septic system. They are a hodgepodge of architectural styles with footprints so large, the development looks more like a Boston neighborhood than rural Carlisle where houses have always had breathing room on their two acres. Each mansion is landscaped with full-grown, ornamental trees and shrubs. Each is surrounded by an antiseptically green lawn devoid of a single dandelion and dotted with underground sprinklers timed to water the lawn even when it's raining.

Recently I read in the local newspaper how the deer population is burgeoning and needs to be controlled to prevent disease and starvation (and damage to expensive landscaping?). I wonder if anyone else questions these conclusions. Of course the deer population is increasing. Other than us they have few predators. Evicted from their homeland by housing developments growing like ubiquitous loosestrife, the deer are forced into ever diminishing patches of habitat.

## ⟋ *February 25*

Today is gray and soaking. I've just returned from taking Hazel to the vet and am greeted by redwing blackbirds singing "cooleege" from the top of the spruce. Softly I call a welcome to them. The cardinals brave the lunch-hour downpour to dine at the feeder outside my office window. The males, bright spots in the hemlock, look like the little scarlet ribbons that decorated the outdoor Christmas tree in December while they watch over their mates cracking sunflower seeds below.

## ⟋ *February 28*

The air is damp and the birds are singing their hearts out. Canada geese are on the move and fly over my head so low, I can hear the rush of air pushing through their flight feathers. The male and his female partner talk to each other in a two-noted honk, which sounds to my ear like one call, but is really one bird answering the other. The lowering sun lights their underbellies and glints off their great, flapping wings as they fly toward the thawing cornfield in search of gleanings. The bachelor geese are looking for mates now and it won't be long before it's time to look for nesting sites among the reeds and marsh grasses down at the bog. There's a lightness in my step this afternoon. I feel taller than usual.

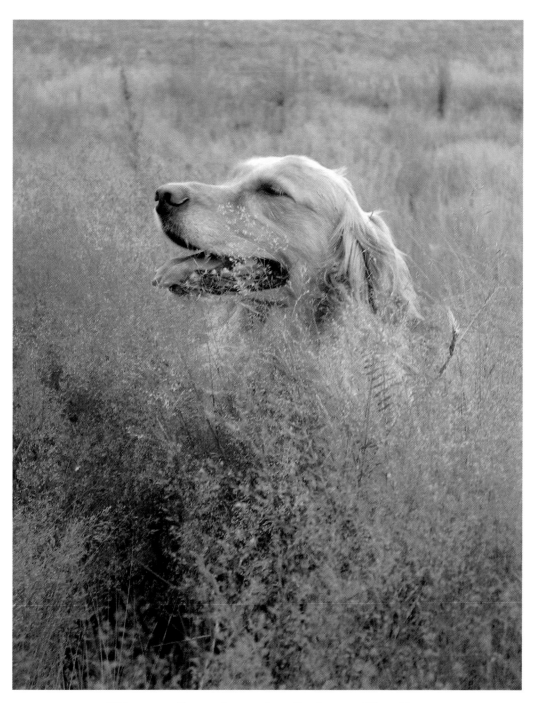

"If you talk to the animals they will talk
with you and you will know each other."
*Chief Dan George*

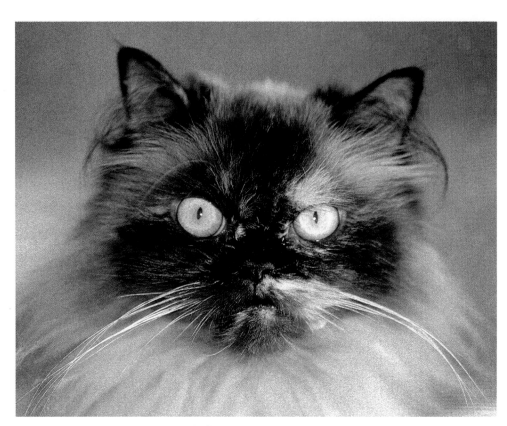

## *The Moment*

The cat sprawls in a sunspot
gazing out the window
at a pair of goldfinches. We listen
to their melancholy chatter.

Green air brushes my skin
I breathe it in and out
and feel a smile
creep in like a flush.

I itch to click my heels.
Suddenly I think,
"I'm happy."

I long to hold on.
But the moment won't bear
the weight of thought.

# Growing Older

At sixty-three, I'm ripe and I've earned the title of "senior." It's a squirmy designation, but the truth be told, I haven't come up with a better one. I'm eligible for any number of trivial and not so trivial discounts offered ripe people; I may buy movie tickets at a child's rate, I have a "golden," fee-less checking account and I get to hear people say, "Gee, I didn't know you were that old, you don't look sixty." The fact is I don't look like what I imagined sixty to look like.

It doesn't seem that long ago I considered sixty over the hill and retreating down the backside—not exactly heading toward heaven. Those were the days when no matter how fast time rushed by, there was an infinite supply of it and its brevity and penchant for running out before I might do the things I wanted, wasn't a concern. So now I have to redefine what being sixty means to me. One thing I know for sure is I've no intention of spending the rest of my life in a perpetual state of mourning the past, yearning for my youth and shuddering at what the future has in store for me. It's not that I think looking back is completely useless. Certainly my follies and indiscretions as well as my triumphs, both large and small, are put in perspective and with a tolerable dose of humility to balance my story I can move inexorably forward into unknown territory.

Growing old isn't easy, especially if one accepts the final outcome as death and after a brush with the possibility of my own extinction, I'm sorely afraid of it. My intelligent self doesn't dispute my terminal existence, but my emotional self says, "Hey, wait a minute, not yet, not yet! And if I should die, let me do it my way, okay?" I'm scared of dying, mostly because I have no idea what it will be like and I can't imagine ceasing to be. How should I make sense of and then peace with the concept of not being? Surely it takes time and endless contemplation. I'm invited by Eastern traditions to "let go" and I'm not sure I'm able to detach in the ways I must to accept either the death of me or of those I love. Such finality is formidable. Accompanying my deep-in-the-belly-fear is another one, no less disturbing. I'm afraid of not having the courage to witness my self perishing little by little should my mind and body parts slowly weaken and fail.

Often when I've ventured to share my fear of recurrent cancer, I'm told, "Well, we're all going to die sometime." I want to scream at the smugness of such a platitude, so glibly declared by someone who's not likely to have examined too closely their own slide toward heaven. The remark is neither compassionate, nor reassuring. It makes me crazy, as does the saying on New Hampshire's license plate, which threatens us all to "live free or die."

But growing older isn't just about endings. No, I don't really like the sags and wrinkles, the stiffening joints and weight gain so difficult these days to control. I surrender to cosmetics, slather myself with moisturizers, curl my hair and feel better when looking my best. I'm not quite at ease with the out-of-my-control changes appearing daily in the mirror. Once in a while I catch my eye in the mirror, make a face at my self and think, "Huh, not so bad." I've got a ways to go before I wear out. In an instant I get how silly it all is and laughter bubbles out of me until I leave the reflection in the glass to get on with my day. I've earned my lines and sooner or later whining gets futile and boring and I realize I'm cheating myself of the pleasure of growing, even if it does mean aging.

Without anxieties and fears I don't think I'd find such delight in moments that now seem extraordinary or in the small joys that accumulate when knowing how fragile is life. Sometimes it feels like I'm practicing to arrive somewhere where I'm not at home—living to the hilt is an enormous challenge. I like to think I'm not done with changing from one skin into another and then another like a dragonfly.

Nowadays, the learning curves are steep and challenging. Learning to be a grandmother, discovering new ways to be a mother and most of all, trying to live with more freedom and passion require energies I didn't know I had. Walls once carefully constructed to protect my vulnerabilities are being chipped away and boundaries long clung to are becoming permeable. Practicing my new voice to say, "I love you" without premeditation when the feeling pops out of somewhere deep inside and free of baggage is as surprising to me as it is satisfying to say, "No, I don't think I want to do that." It's as if making it through sixty years accords me the privilege of speaking out of my heart with less censorship than my head is used to. I can be delighted and frightened, confused and clear, anxious and bold, angry and depressed and know that I have choices. I can choose to do what scares me and survive.

So here I am growing older in this early dawn. One last evening star blinks and is quickly extinguished as the sky transforms itself from deep blue-gray to pale blue. My neighborhood still sleeps. I can hear the distant call of a Canada goose as she rouses her sleeping flock over in the cornfield. Rosie sprawls full length along my side, warming me in the chilly morning air. Patches puddles herself on top of the pillow above my head like a furry nightcap. We three breathe together.

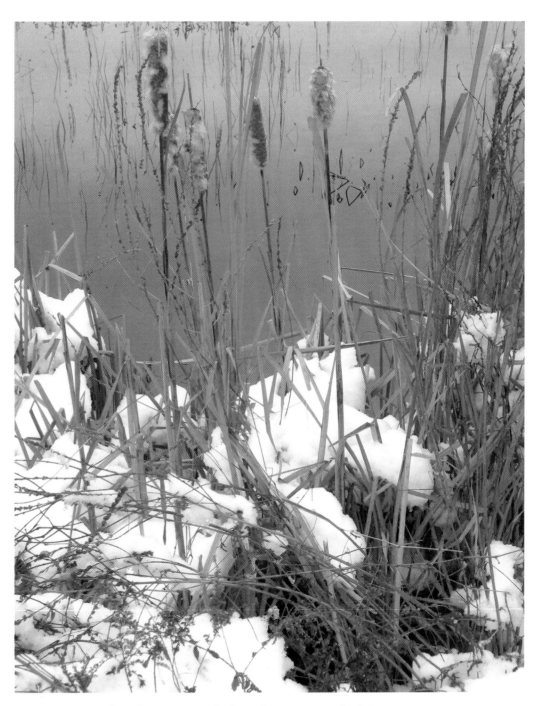

"To know one's landscape, to feel in sympathy with it, is often to be at peace with life."

*Richard E. Dodge*

# March

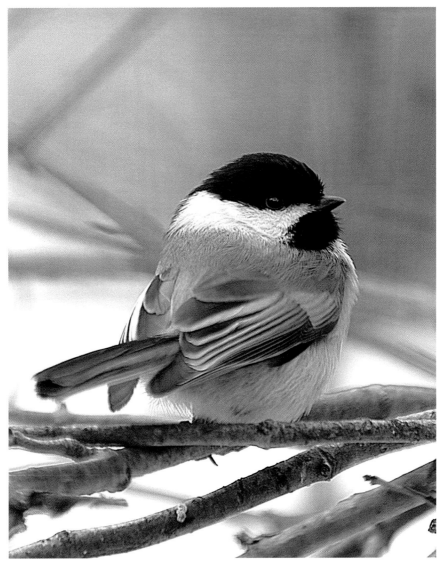

"If you want to see birds, you must have birds in your heart."

*John Burroughs*

# March Journal

## March 3

Clumps of silver clouds plod eastward revealing a pale sun bright enough to let me cast a shadow. The birds fill the air with songs.

A tiny brown bird came to my window feeder singing an insistent and lovely melody. I hadn't seen our Carolina wren for a few weeks and there he was. The recent warmth and rain have been with us until last night's frigid air, which has left the dripping neighborhood looking like a jewelry box filled with sparkling weeds and twigs and grasses hung with crystal drops.

In the woods, the pines sing and shake off thin layers of ice like shards of tinkling glass. The dome of the sky has turned deep blue and is crowded with bundles of puffy clouds. High above us three red-tailed hawks spiral around powerful updrafts. I think they're courting—the female being pursued and impressed by the acrobatics of her two suitors.

All of a sudden out of the west an enormous blanket of charcoal-bellied clouds sweeps over us and obliterates the sun. The wind becomes a gale flinging snowflakes so thick I can barely see a few feet in front of me. The birds go silent and only a solitary, obstreperous crow protests the weather change. As quickly as they came, the clouds disappear into the eastern horizon and a cascade of sunlight pours warmth over the cranberry meadow and dissolves the snow dust. Then it happens all over again—out of nowhere the sky turns to lead and the wind blows icy and thick with snow. Rosie's ears are flying and I huddle again into the collar of my jacket marveling at the fierceness of these fitful storms.

## March 16

An hour before daybreak and all's quiet except for what sounds like white noise— a tuneless, wordless hum. Listening carefully I realize it's the sound of the distant grid of highways, which snake through the landscape to the north and west of my house and the westerly wind is carrying the hum my way. Lying here in bed I envision a streaming river of light as the morning traffic builds and engines roar down the wind into my ears like blood whooshing through the arteries behind my ears. Often I'm not aware of this white noise because I'm tuned into more harmonious sounds close by. A breeze whooshing through the tall evergreens around the house sucks up the hum or a flock of sparrows chatting or a neighbor's dog barking eliminates the incessant background noise. Once in a while I hear the roll and whistle of a train traveling west out of Boston to Fitchburgh as it passes over railway crossings with ill-lit coaches carrying one or two passengers home or away. The whistle pierces the air with a lonesome wail. And I don't mind the occasional roar of a jet passing overhead winking red and green wing-lights—it's the white noise and dirt pollution that irritate me.

Years ago I puzzled over the thin film of gritty dust that coated everything inside my house when I opened the windows for fresh country air. Then I knew the wind not only carried sound, it blew particles of exhaust and road dirt hovering over the highways through my windows. Invisible dust clouds drift over meadows and fallow fields, are trapped by millions of evergreen needles and tree leaves until they sift into a fine, dark grit, which settles over everything—even dulling the iridescent blue of an iris petal, fading the new shine of spring leaves and collecting on my window sills. Still, the air smells clean and when the sky is very blue, I'm unaware of the invisible motes hitching a ride on the west wind.

## March 17

Yesterday felt like May. It brought a light breeze whose little gusts kissed my face and lifted my hair as I walked along the dike trail with Rosie. Today the snow is flying. The birds are confused and so am I. The maples and birches their swollen buds waiting to burst open, have shriveled against the cold. So much weather, so New England, I don't think I could live in a place less challenging. New England's capricious climate forces you to be flexible, inventive and hardy, and you can always talk about the weather when you've nothing else to say.

Female redwing blackbirds have finally arrived and the neighborhood rings with mating calls as the dapper, red-shouldered males argue noisily over territory and mates in the branches of the maple in front of the house. I delight in their gabbing until there's an abrupt and total silence. It's as if an invisible conductor has signaled his orchestra to rest the music or perhaps they've seen a predator. Not a sound—then the exuberant chatter begins again. It reminds me of the erratic snow squalls a few days ago.

Just outside the open window, perched on a dogwood twig, is a lone, small brown-streaked sparrow-sized bird warbling to himself so faintly I can barely make out his lilting song. I wonder if he's a song sparrow arrived too early and confused by the vagaries of our weather.

During the past few days a solitary chickadee comes to the feeder closest to the porch keeping on the outskirts of the resident flock. One foot hangs useless and to eat a sunflower seed, he must hold it with the toes of his good foot while at the same time grasping the twig to stay upright. Such courage in such a tiny creature. What will happen to him? So far, he seems quite able to get enough seeds during lulls at the feeders.

The courting season is in full swing in my neighborhood and down at the bog. Flocks of chickadees have broken up into pairs and titmice sing "chiva-chiva-chiva" to prospective brides. No longer do these gregarious little birds congregate in large numbers at the feeders. Male goldfinches molting into their lemon-yellow plumage are bright as daffodils, although some haven't completely changed and still look shabby. Red and gray squirrels chase each other spiraling around and up and down tree trunks, chittering noisily as they race across the snow and up another tree. They're so preoccupied; they don't seem at all interested in raiding the feeding stations.

Listening to the busyness outside my window reminds me how much I love this season of births and beginnings and how I too, await a birth. My daughter-in-law looks radiant and ponderously uncomfortable with her hard belly stretched to its limit in this her last pregnant month. She tells me the baby is very active and appears to know her own mind even in the womb. I remember when long ago and in the same state of expectancy, I was certain my belly skin would burst if the child I carried dawdled any longer.

## March 18

A last dusting of snow has cleaned up our dingy, leaf-littered lawn. This afternoon Barry and I took the dogs to explore the Estabrook Woods, hoping to follow its long trail for a short way. The head of the trail led into a hardwood forest where the ground beneath the trees was clear of undergrowth and saplings. In spite of the snow the trail was easy to walk and the soft crunch of our footfalls lured us further and further into the woods until we came to a fork in the trail and decided to "take the one less traveled." Here the hardwoods gave way to a large stand of ancient hemlocks with long, slender, arms drooping to the ground. We trudged on until we finally came to an opening in the forest and found ourselves at the foot of Punkatasset Hill, a small hillock, which as a child, I thought was huge, especially when I hauled my toboggan all the way to the top. Beneath the hill is Punkatasset Pond, another childhood haunt. When no one had swimming pools, this was our swimming hole on hot summer afternoons. It didn't matter there were giant snapping turtles napping in the bottom mud. I didn't care. The coppery water was even cool enough to entice my mother to splash with me.

Stubborn about retracing steps, I voted for continuing down Monument Street in search of the proper trail end off Estabrook Road, which I knew wasn't too far off. The walk was considerably longer than I'd expected and by the time the four of us headed back up the trail to Carlisle, we were panting with exertion. The estimated half hour walk had turned into two magical hours of walking on fresh snow into the silent woods. I suspect this will be the last snowfall of the season.

## March 23

The birches are twitching with catkins and halfway around the cranberry meadow, the voices of a pair of spring peepers are tuning up and bluebirds softly twitter deep in a trailside thicket. I can see neither the little frogs nor the elusive birds.

The small ditches lining the edge of the meadow are clogged with thick green goo, which holds masses of frog's eggs—minuscule black dots encased in jelly. As a child I filled mason jars with frog jelly and spent days watching the eggs hatch into polliwogs with tails. In time, the tails disappeared and miniature legs grew out of the infant tadpole's bellies and if I were lucky the jar filled with baby frogs, which I dumped back into the swamp, but more often the contents of the jar turned rancid, much to my disappointment, and had to be flushed down the toilet.

As Rosie and I round the corner by the large pond where stacks of beehives have stood dormant for so many months, some crazy honeybees attack us. Dozens of them dive-bomb my head and chase us both down the path, stinging us wherever they chance to find bare skin. I've never seen unprovoked bees so angry. I hope they're in a better mood tomorrow. We finish our walk.

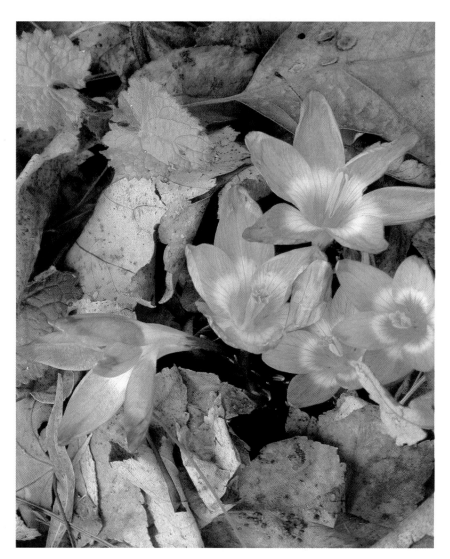

## *March*

Out of the moldering litter,
polished with arrows of sun,
tentative swellings prick
the garden's bare and icy skin.

A docile wind tickles boughs of hemlock
stiff with rime. It ruffles my hair.
The air is thick with exuberant voices.
I want to sing my carol
with the bluebirds, titmice and sparrows,
and coax a purple crocus into bloom.

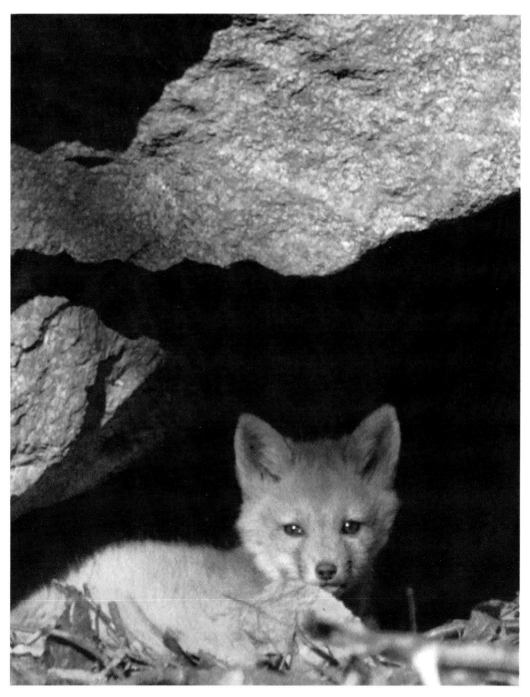

"With all beings and all things we shall
be as relatives."

*Black Elk*

# Thoughts on the Wind

"The oldest voice in the world is the
wind."
*Donald Culross Peattie (1898–1964)*

Lately, I've become aware of air all around me. I've never thought much about the wind until now. Excepting the most obvious impact of wind, both gentle and harsh, it either cooled me off in summer or bit me in winter. It began with dancing flowers, which I struggled to render in sharp detail with my camera. As soon as I carefully focused my lens on a blossom, it softly swayed out of focus and I ended up with a wastebasket full of blurry photographs. After studying the situation I grasped what was happening. The smallest breeze invites flowers to toss their heads, but every now and again the breeze holds its breath and I hold mine and the blossoms stop nodding long enough for me to capture a sharp image.

The wind touches all of my senses. I can see the wind make a field of grass undulate like ocean surf or clouds roll like billowing sails across the sky. I've seen enormous trees bend to a gale just as I'm forced to lean into a blustery northwest wind just to make headway along the bog trail. Long ago in the midst of a September hurricane, I remember sneaking barefoot out of our battened-down house, curious to feel the might of the wind and the thrust of warm rain slanting against my face. My beloved elm creaked and groaned as the gale tore off its leaves and branches and a row of hemlocks, ringing our house, bowed to the ground and sprung back until one cracked in two. Nearby, the brook had exploded with froth and overran its banks.

Charged with the energy of the storm raging around me and oblivious to its danger, I felt reckless and free. Not until night approached and the steely sky turned a formidable black, not until I watched the one streetlight at the end of the driveway flicker and go out, did I return home to the angry dismay of my mother, who'd lost me.

When the first gentle wind of spring whispers confidences in my ear and riffles my hair like a lover, my heart skips and I fly with the bell song of a bobolink on its invisible currents. The smallest breath ripples the surface of the bog pond into designs not unlike those it carves in desert sands. I've been drenched by salt spray blown from the tops of in-rushing waves and watched the wind compel these waves into breakers that devour the shore. When it whistles through door cracks and makes windows shudder, it's mysterious and spine tingling. In spring clouds of pollen are borne on the wind to dust the landscape yellow. Silky seed filaments of dandelions and milkweed drift on the wind and spores and microscopic seeds are blown to fertile resting places.

Wind makes wonderful sounds—like the creaking of windmills pulling water from the earth or the clatter of whirligigs sawing logs on a garden fence or the chatter of spinning pinwheels. I'd like to be lifted off my feet and drift on the wind's silent currents like a glider or a hawk. Frightening winds may blow into a tornado and level a village and I've heard if a long wind sweeps across a prairie for days and days, it can drive people crazy. Polluted air borne on the wind mixes with rain to form toxic acids, which kill fish in lakes and ponds.

Wind pushes weather along a prevailing course. Like water, it flows in currents and like water if it meets an obstacle, it may arbitrarily shift its direction to bring a sudden change in the forecast. Scores of names describe the many faces and personalities of the wind: There are headwinds, tail winds and trade winds, sea breezes, land breezes, westerlies and polar easterlies. There are whirlwinds, jet streams and gales, hurricanes, tornadoes and wet monsoons. In France a mistral blows chilly squalls out of the Rhone Valley. Warm foehns tumble down Alpine slopes much like the Chinooks, which blow out of Canada onto the eastern Rocky Mountains. The hot, dry sirocco winds sear the land near the Mediterranean and blue-northers buffet the western United States. Noreasters bring rain or snow to New England.

I know physics has something to do with the wind's behavior; our rotating earth, its sun, the creation of gases, the rising of hot air, the descent of cold air, all conspire to produce wind currents and build pressure systems that spawn weather. When I watch the wind paint sunset clouds in orange, pink and lavender on a sky-blue canvas, I'm astonished every time it happens, even though I'm aware the wind's flung billions of microscopic particles into the atmosphere to catch the last blaze of sun slouching toward the horizon. And when I think the show is done, when the sun's disappeared, the wind splashes even more brilliant colors across the horizon. The wind sculpts clouds into all manner of shapes: Mackerel clouds, horsetails, billows of puffy clouds, black-bellied clouds, towers and bunches of clouds and I'm enchanted when I discover faces, shapes of animals fashioned out of clouds by this amazing artist. These days I relish its soft breath in my ear, its kiss on my face, its bite and chill, which bring tears to my eyes and now with the wind at my back nudging me along the bog trail, my thoughts rise with a red-tailed hawk spiraling on invisible eddies.

# Wind in the Leaves

A child watches scarlet leaves
riffle along a bough, skipping
to their own soughing music
and she wonders.
Who's stuck them on their twigs?
Who makes them turn and dance?
Do flying leaves compel the wind
to whisper in her ear?

When the child is gone and winter comes,
when all the leaves have come unglued
and ice-rimed branches clink together
where promises keep and flowers rest,
she'll come again to wonder
what it is that's made them sing.

# April

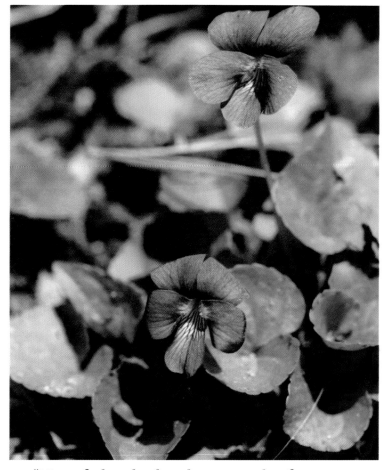

"Now fades the last long streak of snow,
Now burgeons every maze of quick
About the flowering squares and thick
By ashen roods the violets blow....
From land to land, and in my breast
Spring wakens too, and my regret
Becomes an April violet,
And buds and blossoms like the rest."

*Alfred Lord Tennyson*

# April Journal

⟋◯ *April 2*

Armed with a picnic basket, blanket and camera, Barry and I drive to Toll's Field. Gus and Rosie are giddy with anticipation of an outing and a ride in the car, if only for a few miles. The weather is mild; a gusty spring breeze freshens the air as we walk across a large open field and into the woods. Searching for a secluded and sheltered spot to picnic, we find a likely place off the trail up a rocky rise. Here we spread the blanket and unleash the dogs to explore the woodsy swamp below our aerie. A splash of sunlight warms the ground beneath us and soaks into the smooth granite boulder that's our backrest. Setting the basket of food aside, Barry settles himself on the blanket with a book and I lean into the warm stone. A tall old pine creaks and sways with the wind, painting patterns across its patch of blue sky where clouds are streaming by. Rosie's been collecting a pile of twigs to chew on and nestles down beside me. Gus mucks about in the swamp. Wagging his tail furiously he sniffs twigs, tufts of grass, pine-cones and tree trunks and then lifts his leg on them.

Deep in the woods the birds are quiet. Perhaps the stiffening wind has discouraged the mating game for the morning. Two frogs croak at each other—first one, then the other answers and both stop when Gus splashes into their little pool of water. A lone chickadee calls out "fee-bee" somewhere in the distance, but there's no answer. So mesmerized by the dancing trees, the music of the wind and the delicious smell of pine needles warming in the April sun, I don't bother to unpack my book or write in the journal as I'd intended.

Barry is hungry and finally rouses himself to set out our lunch of hard-boiled eggs, tuna salad, tabouli, fresh strawberries with cupcakes and a bottle of wine. Smelling the food, I'm suddenly famished. It's perfect: This wind-touched place, the sun gilding the wine, the strawberries, the smell of spring woods and the happy dogs rustling in the leaf litter. Neither of us speak, as if in silent agreement not to disturb the moment. When we've finished eating, I take out my camera and join the dogs to explore the site for photo opportunities. A skunk cabbage, sunlight glowing in its unfurling, veined leaves, catches my eye and tickles my nose. Hiding in a mottled green and purple spathe, spring's first flower sends its skunky perfume to entice a pollinator. I'm reminded of long ago Aprils when, as a child, I splashed through swampy places looking for frog's eggs and other spring treasures. Then I stumble on a collage of pinecones, needles, brittle oak leaves and a tiny, green mound of wild violets with tight buds curled amidst heart-shaped leaves.

It's gotten late and time to leave. We pack up our things, leash the panting dogs and head home. There's still time to have a bog walk. The late afternoon wind carves blue and black ripples across the surface of the pond. Armed with my camera I'd hoped to photograph maple flowers and seeds backlit by the lowering sun against the blue sky, but the wind prevents me. These days the sun is setting even later than I've remembered in the past. As usual, daylight savings probably confuses me.

The past week sped by so quickly and with the exception of an attack of moodiness, it was a good one. Tonight has brought a long-awaited gift. At 9:24 P.M. my granddaughter was born, causing some concern as she pushed into the world clutching her umbilical cord. She came quickly, in any case, and is a robust little creature with lots of dark hair. I'm a nana.

## April 3

I'm infused with energy this morning and have decided to take Rosie on a long walk around Great Meadows Refuge in Concord. Becoming a grandmother has transformed me and put an extra bounce in my step as we hike the circumference of the marsh and the pond where Rosie spots a river otter floating on his back holding a morsel of something in his paws. He eyes us, unperturbed by our proximity, and I delight in this cocky, playful creature, who rolls over and slips away when he's finished eating. The meadow teems with birds—mostly waterfowl: Ducks and Canada geese float on the pond flipping their rears into the air as they dip beneath the surface to graze. A great blue heron, barely visible, stands among the tall reeds sprouting out of last year's dead stalks. The redwings are ubiquitous as are sparrows; tiny warblers just arriving from the south flit in and out of newly blossoming trees. On the way home, three wild turkey hens poke out of a thicket beside the road to scratch in the gravel.

In celebration of birth and spring, my house is filled with flowers. A bouquet of yellow roses, pink tulips and lavender anemones sits on my writing table in the porch where pots of Easter lilies, purple hyacinths and pink and blue hydrangeas line the sills and baskets of fern hang from the ceiling. I'm off to the hospital to hold Ilaria Agassiz Fordyce.

A white cap covers her copious hair and she's swaddled in a soft blanket. Ilaria's fingers are long and perfect and she's got delicately shaped eyebrows and a Cupid's bow mouth—lovely like her mother's. It's astonishing how this birth has affected me. I'm exhilarated, inspired and elated all at once, and I keep saying her name, "Ilaria" to myself over and over like a mantra. Her father is large with pride and her mother, though wan with exhaustion, looks as beatified as a Renaissance Madonna. She'd giggle at this hyperbole.

## April 5

I was awakened this morning by the intense and ardent clamor of birdsong. They've sung ceaselessly since sunrise. Now the symphony seems to have climaxed and I suspect the birds are busy with foraging and housekeeping. I'm still having difficulty recognizing more than a few individual calls in spite of listening to the birdsong CD over and over. The morning is warm and a small breeze drifts through my open window.

Down at the bog the swamp maples are in bloom and their blushing flowers tint the landscape soft pink. The red-tailed hawk glides with his mate over the bog meadows playing with the wind currents. Closer to earth frogs croak, trill, grunt and chirp, their cacophonous music. Big green frogs pluck banjoes while sunning beside a murky ditch and plop into the water when Rosie and I walk by. Now and again a bullfrog utters a guttural "chug-a-rum" from somewhere deep in the reeds. In vernal pools tadpoles are hatching even as their unconcerned parents sing their hearts out from the trees or from within the masses of cat-o'-nine-tails just spiking up through the bog muck and turning green.

At midday I drove to the city to have lunch with my son, my daughter-in-law and my granddaughter, who's now five days old. I got to hold her and change her diaper, which I hadn't done in over thirty years, but what mother forgets how to diaper a baby? My son was quick to point out I'd put Ilaria's Pamper on backward. I trust grandmothering will be easier than mothering. As I was photographing her, this little creature opened her blue eyes and I could swear she smiled.

This evening Barry came home from work early in time for a dusky walk to the bog. Overcome with excitement at this unexpected outing and in spite of my sharp remonstrance, Rosie plunged into the blackest, muddiest ditch she could find. When she finally heeded my call, she trotted toward me looking more like a Labrador retriever than a golden. I was furious and gave her a good scolding after which she spent the next ten minutes walking as close to my legs as possible, smearing my jeans with oily mud. I think she hoped to make up for her transgression by heeling without being told. At the edge of the upper pond we stopped by a shallow, sandy spot where a reluctant Rosie was forced to take a deep, long swim to wash off the slime. At dusk tree swallows dove through the air around us as we turned toward home.

I was eight when I discovered barn swallows living in our cow barn. Families of iridescently blue-black birds returned each spring to build their mud and grass nests high up in the hand-hewn rafters of the hayloft. In and out they zoomed through chinks in the eaves. I'd climb up the long wooden ladder into the loft and stand precariously on a wobbly pile of hay bales to see into the nests. Most were situated so high I'd have to reach my hand up to feel for tiny eggs or squirmy little hatchlings. I remember how hot and stuffy the loft was and how hay dust glittered in the shafts of sunlight coming through the window in the roof's peak as the squeaking swallows, alarmed by my egregious intrusion, dove at my head, keeping up their heroic attack until I aborted my mission, climbed down the ladder and left the barn.

Occasionally I plucked a lovely aqua egg from a nest to take home to add to my collection of birds' nests, eggshells and found-feathers. In those days my curiosity was insatiable and I filched from nature whatever caught my imagination. Not only did I rob birds' nests, I picked and pressed fragile wildflowers between pages of my mother's books, or chased elusive monarchs and swallowtails with a butterfly net. Once caught, they were mercilessly killed with a cotton ball daubed in chloroform in a mason jar. Then the "specimen" was mounted on cotton-batting and covered with a glass frame. These acts of wanton thievery weren't so different from those of my ancestors who had an even greater penchant for collecting long before technology made it possible to observe wild creatures in their natural habitat without harming them.

At some point my acquisitiveness turned into compassion and I armed myself with notebooks and pencils and aided by Golden Nature Guides, I collected observations instead of wild things. Now I collect their images on film. A stream of delicious memories like these bring back careless summer days spent in the meadows and forests flanking my home, indulging a passionate desire to learn. Later an equally passionate love of animals sustained the feisty teenager I became who plunged headfirst and kicking into adulthood. My horse listened patiently, ears pricked forward, she nuzzled me gently when I hung on her neck crying out my woeful tales and my golden dog licked away the tears.

## April 14

I would have slept in this morning had Rosie not breathed so heavily in my ear. We play an odd game, she and I. She exhales a whoosh of air and I match her breath for breath. She stops briefly, I do too—and we begin to breathe together all over again. I wonder if she's aware of playing this breathing game with me?

A walk at high noon. Way up in the branches of a flowering red maple I spot a minuscule nest clinging to two twigs hanging over the trail. It can't be more than three inches in diameter. The wonder is with all my careful attention passing by this tree so often, I've never seen the little nest, which today holds fast to its crutch of twigs in spite of a gusty April wind. My fantasy lifts me into the nest and I feel like the child in the Mother Goose lullaby who's warned, "Hush-a-bye-baby, on the tree top! When the wind blows the cradle will rock; when the bough breaks, the cradle will fall; down will come baby, bough, cradle and all." I'm almost certain this nest belonged to a goldfinch family whose tiny hatchlings rocked in the wind as precariously as my imagination does today. Goldfinches like to build their nests twenty feet above the earth, unlike sparrows and warblers who prefer to make theirs closer to terra firma.

At home I'm consumed by a restless urge to start the book I've wanted to write for so long. I can think of nothing to stop me from facing this dreaded dream head-on. As anxious as I am to begin, I'm terrified of getting discouraged and losing interest. Dissatisfied with past efforts, pages of unfinished material collected in notebooks and in wastebaskets, material I once thought interesting, but later found boring and fatuous. This time I'm determined to stick with it notwithstanding the insistent, belittling voice that shouts that it's a vain conceit to even think I might write a book of interest to anyone. Writing here helps me set a course.

## April 16

The air is heavy with moisture, but in spite of its oppressive thickness, walking the bog trails is refreshing. As always it's a treat for Rosie. The meadows ring with the songs of white-throated sparrows, song sparrows, warblers, killdeer, Canada geese and frogs. Pairs of mallards skim the ditches on squeaky wings looking for a place to land and a flock of geese wings over the meadow and sets down on the pond where they form a raft of tranquil, preening birds. All of a sudden, one goose begins to honk until the whole crowd joins in. Then as if on some mysterious signal, with the wind at its back, the flock flaps into the air heading to the cornfield where a green beard of succulent grass has sprouted. I love to watch geese flying on a windy day. They twist and turn in the air, executing aerobatic rolls until they near the water where they land with outstretched necks and legs splayed out in front like brakes. Pushing the black water with webbed feet, the geese coast across its surface like so many water-skiers.

A small painted turtle has pulled itself out of the pond with its long toenails and slowly inches its way into the woods. I follow a Lilliputian blue butterfly dipping in the breeze hoping it'll land nearby. It disappears. Dandelions are in full bloom and clumps of bluets dot the banks of the ditches. At home our pear tree blooms with a cloud of honeybees humming in its flower-filled branches. They flit from blossom to blossom, sipping nectar until the little bags of pollen on their legs are full enough to return to the hive.

This afternoon driving home from town, I saw a red fox saunter out of a thicket beside the road. He trotted casually in front of my car and stopped. I stopped. He hesitated and looked me square in the eye. I looked back at him, surprised by his audacity. When he was ready, he ambled across the cornfield and disappeared into a stand of pines at the far end. With a lingering sense of amazement at the encounter I continued toward home and had to stop again when four deer, who'd been grazing a neighbor's lawn, stepped daintily across the road in front of me. They too vanished into the woods.

## April 18

I feel light and happy to be alive today. The afternoon is blue. It glows with sunshine until a scrim of clouds sneaks in on a westerly breeze and bleaches the sky. Most of the hardwood trees are in full bloom. Oaks and maples, elms and birches have transformed the landscape with lovely, pale-green tints. It will be a while yet before the evergreens throw their extravagant sacks of pollen dust over everything.

Walking beside the bog pond, I look up to see two large birds soaring above the water, each in opposite corners so high as to be almost invisible in the blue air. I stop to watch their odd behavior; The larger of the two black birds circles higher, then hovers briefly, beating the air slowly until suddenly it pulls its wings into the shape of a trident and plummets headfirst out of the sky and into the pond with a large splash. The bird surfaces flapping its powerful wings and rises into the air with a large fish in its talons. I can hardly believe my eyes; it's an osprey. I've never seen any away from the coast of Maine.

I watch the pair of osprey until they disappear over the tops of the pine trees. Also known as fish hawks, these birds are the only raptor to dive for fish and only eagles are larger than these handsome birds. I've read that an osprey clings so fiercely to its prey that even if the fish is too heavy to haul from the water the bird will drown before it lets go. Now that's either stupid, stubborn or desperate. Their courtship is a sight I'd love to witness and perhaps have, unwittingly, since the two now dancing over the bog pond are male and female, she being the larger of the two birds. I can just make out the male's high-pitched shrieks as he soars and swoops around the object of his love. Ospreys are known to build their nests inland in a dead treetop sturdy enough to hold the weight of a branch-and-stick structure five feet around and up to seven feet high. Such an enormous nest is hard to imagine. I hope this pair stays with us for a while.

## April 22

I woke this morning grumpy with stiffness. I worry these sore joints will only worsen with age. The fact is, last night sleep was fitful at best because of the monotonous pounding of rain and a disagreeable cold prickling my nose. I think I understand the concept of weather cells. In the middle of the night, dazzling slashes of lightning lit up the porch announcing a single, colossal thunder boom, which shook the walls. A long silence followed, broken only by rain spitting on the sky window. Just when I dozed off to sleep, another flash, another ear-splitting crack, and this time, pounding rain battered the roof until another storm came through. These storms came in short bursts and made me think of weather cells as they passed to the east over and over again, unlike an ordinary thunderstorm, which comes in from a distance, rages and weakens as it moves out of the neighborhood.

Heavily dosed with Echinacea, black elderberry syrup and double doses of vitamin C throughout the day, my cold has been nipped in the bud and I'm able to settle down to write in my journal and work on the book. There I said it, "the book." Rosie lies on my foot sound asleep. From where I sit, I can see the top of the spruce tree where two forbidding, old crows cackle at one another and watch the cardinals below vie for a place at the feeder with cowbirds, blue jays and a flock of redwings. It's almost time for tea at the end of a peaceful, meandering day in which a bit of creative effort has proved a tonic to my spirits as much as the disappearing cold has done.

### April 28

Today is my solo in the woods. The morning has brought sun and a gentle breeze just enough to blow insects away. I'm prepared to spend the day alone without Rosie. Waking early, I pull on my jeans and a T-shirt, tie a windbreaker around my waist, and stuff a backpack with a lean picnic of cheese, crackers, a tin of peaches, a bottle of water, my camera, a notebook, pen and pencil, a jackknife and a space blanket.

### 7:45 A.M.

Walking past the bog pond and into the woods, I already wish I'd brought Rosie to keep me company. Dismissing my fear of becoming a victim of human mischief in a dark forest, I head toward the large pine, which marks where I leave the trail through the thick underbrush into a small patch of wilderness where my secret spot is encircled with stones I've collected over the last weeks. I rake away twigs and woody debris with my fingers and spread the space blanket over a thin mattress of pine needles. I'm sweating by the time I finish making a suitable nest for myself. There are no signs of life in the beaver hut in front of my circle and I'd hoped to see one. Two male Canada geese glide in and around the grass hummocks rising out of the black swamp water. They eye me with curiosity. I suspect they're patrolling nearby where their mates sit on carefully concealed nests among the cattails. Normally vocal, they make their rounds in silence intent on decoying predators away from the area.

### 8:30 A.M.

The sun covers me with comfortable warmth and I'm happy within my stone circle, except for a not-unexpected touch of restlessness. Pushing my backpack into a pillow and stuffing it under my head, I look up through a filigree of pine branches into the chicory sky. Millions of shiny green needles stir in the air above me where a flutter of wings brings a raccoon-faced common yellow-throated warbler and his mate to play among the pine twigs. She plays hard to get as he chases her from branch to branch. A bright yellow warbler joins the courting pair, swings for a moment on a twig and is off with a twitter. Out on the swamp redwings flash their epaulets from the tips of last year's reeds where new green shoots are poking out of the water. A large, fat bumblebee has come to rest on my notebook until it realizes I'm me and zooms angrily away. A great blue heron flaps across the distant sky just above a stand of maples whose blushing new leaves make a lovely display of pink, pale red, pastel greens and fawn colors. The heron becomes a speck on the horizon.

### 9:00 A.M.

Just as I begin to doze off, I'm aroused by the melancholic greeting of a pair of goldfinches who swoop across the marsh toward me. Landing on the branch vacated by the warblers, they talk in soft voices. Then deep in the woods a flicker squawks, startling the little birds, who fly away calling to one another as if to reassure themselves no one is chasing them. The flicker continues to drill noisily for his mate. The sky has suddenly changed its disposition. The wind freshens and feels cool on my arms and clouds sweep in from the northwest.

### 10:30 A.M.

I've had to put on my jacket now that darkly ominous clouds have obliterated the sun and only a few patches of blue sky remain. This wasn't in the forecast, but I should know better than to put much stock in the weather people, who in spite of their fancy technology can't seem to predict the vagaries of New England weather any more accurately than does *The Farmer's Almanac*. The wind is chilly and I've had to wrap the space blanket around me to stay warm. To keep occupied I'm trying to distinguish one bird's song from another with limited success. From a nearby thicket bordering the swamp, mourning doves coo their dolorous songs. A pair flies on squeaky wings to the branch above my head landing heavily on this popular twig causing it to bow and dip. I pray they don't mess on me. Where the marsh opens into the bog pond, a swarm of swallows flits low over the water looking for newly hatched flies. When the intensifying wind frustrates their efforts, they vanish into the woods. I'm grateful not to have to fend off voracious insects this morning.

### 11:30 A.M.

The clouds have completely filled the sky and a sprinkle of rain spits on the space blanket. The wind is raw and cold and my fingers are so stiff it's hard to hold a pen to write. I wonder if I'll be able to stick it out here. This stinks!

### 1:30 P.M.

The spitting rain has moved off and a few hopeful breaks open in the cloud cover, but the bone-chilling wind remains. I'm hungry and form the space blanket into a facsimile of a tent using my sitting body as a tent pole, while I fasten the corner grommets with elastic bands to keep the ends from flapping. I'm beginning to feel adventurous instead of a miserable victim of the weather as I dig into the goat cheese and crackers. The tin of peaches tastes wonderful! Halfway through a meager but truly satisfying lunch, the rain starts again, but I decide to stay a while longer. It'll be okay so long as I keep dry, if not completely warm. Like me the smaller birds have taken shelter and except for crows and geese, who continue to go about their business unfazed by the wind, there's no activity around me.

### ∾ 3:30 P.M.

Ah! A blue patch of sky has opened up and a spray of sunlight warms me. I need to stretch my cramped body and so uncocoon myself. It amazes me how the wind softens and dies when the sun catapults from behind the clouds, then swaggers again as the sun becomes shrouded by a new army of clouds. The wind has been the star of the day, but I'm praying it calms down now I've decided to step out of the circle of stones with my camera to explore the woods.

Large rocks dressed in mounds of velvety green mosses with miniature ferns sprouting out of them lay along the banks of the marsh. I'm not sure film will capture the softness of the mosses and the delicacy of the ferns against the hard gray rock or do justice to the coarse texture of wet pine bark, or to the deepening shadows cast by the afternoon sun. Hoping to stumble on a wild creature, I'm lured further into the wild underbrush where the birds have joyfully resumed their singing.

### ∾ 5:30 P.M.

It's time to go home. I've stayed as long as I'd planned and feel satisfied with myself for sticking it out. With my gear packed away, I make my way back onto the woods trail and head toward the bog pond. The air is considerably warmer, not yet balmy, but sedate and the bright sun dips toward a clear horizon. I'm starving and eager to be taken out for a scrumptious dinner.

### ∾ April 29

This morning I woke up drained of yesterday's positive energy. A black mood has sucked the sun right out of the blue sky suddenly and without warning. That this happens at all is disappointing and I'm angry thinking how hard I've worked to shore up my spiritual center and free it from depressing ghosts, which so easily tug me into old shadowy corners. I remind myself that spring heralds not just joy and excitement, but these days an anniversary reaction to the time seven springs ago when I was pitched face-to-face with my mortality with a diagnosis of breast cancer. I'd hoped these feelings would ameliorate with time. Am I more susceptible to these anxieties than other survivors?

In this mood tumultuous thoughts come unbidden: how to be a grandmother. If I had a model it would be my nana, whose unconditional love for me remains the essence of what I want to bring to my granddaughter. While I've struggled not to repeat my mother's shortcomings, in the past I somehow managed to make my own worse with the effort, always afraid I'll lose her in my heart as I reinvent my own roles as mother and grandmother. With angry intensity, both my adult children have brought to my attention old wounds and resentments about my unacceptable mothering. Right or wrong, distorted or not, I've been helpless to make their pain go away, either by acknowledging it or by apologizing for my shortcomings. After several painful years of estrangement, each of my children has become willing to engage in a healing process with me. For my part, I've learned to let go of unsuccessful habits of interacting with each one. I've let go of unreasonable expectations about how I thought we'd relate together when we all became adults. I have control over so little and yet so much of my self is controlled by old history and my perceptions, it's hard always to know what to keep and what to let go of, especially for a tenacious collector like me. Why shouldn't the birth of a granddaughter be unaccompanied by such angst and bring only delight? I remind myself I've been here before and this sudden squall of reverie will abate as quickly as it appeared. In the meantime I hunker down into the sofa under the cover of sunlight coming through the sky window and distract myself with a good book until the mood lifts.

It's been a strange day. Afternoon clouds roll in to block the sun just when my dark thoughts begin to drift off, thoughts as tenacious and as capricious as the wind pushing these billows. Barry and I walk the dogs to the bog where our shadows are visible when the sun nudges through a blue hole in the clouds. We walk in silence broken only when we spot a female American kestrel, not much larger than a blue jay, brave the stiff breeze and flap low over the meadow scanning for mice. For now my mind floods with peace.

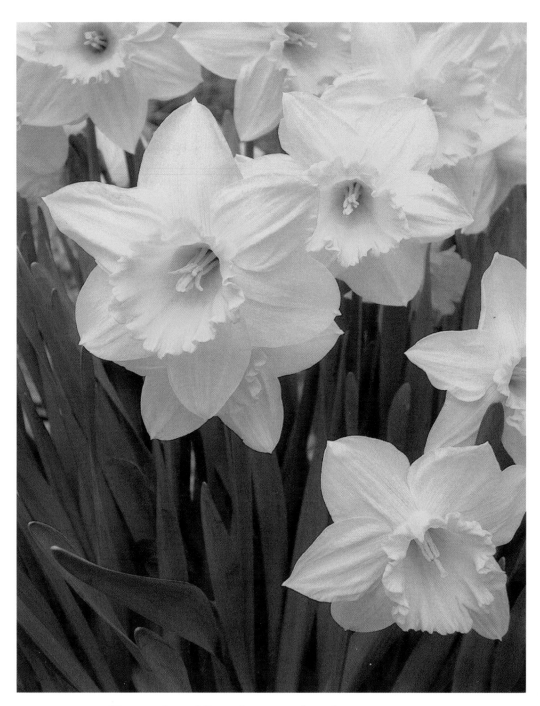

"I wandered lonely as a cloud
That floats on high o'er vales and hills.
When all at once I saw a crowd,
A host of golden daffodils…"

*William Wordsworth*

# Owl

High in the loft
on a shadowy beam
moon-eyes blink
at a drizzle of sun, the owl
swings her head, probes stale corners
where spiders fling their webs.

When the dusky light flickers out
she shrieks into the night
on soft and noiseless wings.

Drowsy mice and I tremble
in our dreams; where the faint memory
of a huntress, her face like a heart,
her talons sharp as knives, preys
on small and feckless souls.

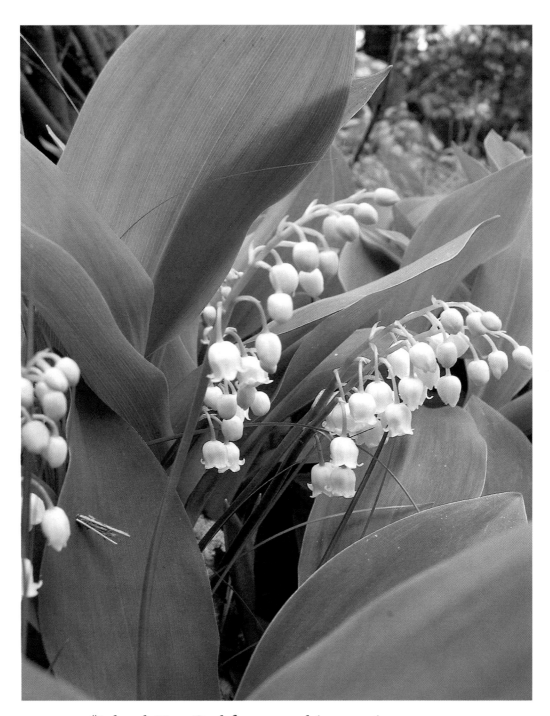

"I thank You God for most this amazing
day: for the leaping greenly spirits of trees
and a blue true dream of sky; and for everything
which is natural which is infinite which is yes."

*e.e. cummings*

# The Story of a Birth

Long ago on a warm summer night a young woman conceived a child. The knowledge filled her with excitement. Shame shrouded the announcement of her child's conception because she had yet to be married but she defied those who would sully her happiness. She felt exquisitely alive. Neither morning sickness nor fatigue interrupted the early months and as the leaves turned to scarlet and yellow, her smooth belly began faintly to swell. On a rainy October afternoon wearing a lovely, ivory wedding dress, her head covered with a fine lace mantilla she'd brought from Spain, she walked proudly down the aisle to marry her husband. Amidst tears of joy they said their vows. Their secret went unnoticed.

After the wedding the young woman drove with her bewildered husband in their tiny car to a city far from home. Here she transformed three small rooms into a nest and began to collect all that she'd need when the baby was born. Remembering how as a little girl she'd loved to play house, how she'd wished then to be grown up just like her mother, all of a sudden she was the grown-up she'd hoped to be: married, with a child growing inside her and not the slightest idea of how to be a wife or a mother. Dreams dreamed long ago embedded in her innermost being unfolded and her life was lit with anticipation. As winter wore on, the child in her dreamed too.

Each day the woman's husband went to work. Alone, she thought about her child. Whatever happened, her child would grow up in a family different from what she'd known. She wanted to be the very best mother. There would be love to spare. She read books—many, many books about how to be a mother, about how babies grew and what they needed at every stage of their development. It was complicated. She wrote endless letters home to her own mother whom she missed very much. When her husband returned to their apartment at night, she fixed him dinner. She wasn't a very good cook because she'd had so little experience. The cook who prepared meals for her family had chased her out of the kitchen when she was working. But the young woman liked to experiment, to be creative, and soon her dinners were palatable.

As she grew in girth there were no baby showers to celebrate the coming child, no one congratulated the almost-mother. Most of the time she forgot how some people thought she'd done something shameful. Instead, she let a sense of wonder fill her. Her mother told her she was sorry but would be far away when it came time for the baby's arrival. That's the way it had to be. The young woman didn't argue, didn't want to deflate the cocoon of happiness she'd built around herself. As the baby grew, she began to feel a whisper deep inside her. At first it felt like a tickle. Then amazingly as her belly grew larger, the tickling of life became a thumping against her taut skin. Each day it seemed her body was transformed, growing larger until finally her navel flattened and disappeared. Once in a while a bump appeared beneath her belly's skin only to melt back into a dark damp place in her womb. Sometimes she would caress the bump. She even began to talk and to sing to her unborn child—this life so uniquely hers for the moment and yet so independent of her all at the same time. Though the young woman marveled at what was happening inside her, sometimes it was frightening and confusing. There was no one she could talk to about such confusing feelings, no one but the doctor whom she saw once a month who reassured her "everything will be all right."

The young woman told her doctor she wanted to be wide awake and present for her baby's birth. The custom of the day was to put a birthing mother into a painless, memory-less sleep from which she would awaken in a white room and wait for her baby to be put into her arms hours after it was born. Long ago, as a girl reading a magazine in a doctor's waiting room, she'd been intrigued by an article about "natural childbirth." In a moment of youthful innocence she vowed to herself that if she ever had a baby, she would know every moment of its coming into the world. The doctor, a kind, fatherly sort of man, agreed that she could be awake when her baby was born, but he demurred when she asked if her husband could be present. The doctor said that if her husband should faint at the sight—as some men must have done—it would distract the nurses and the doctor who, then, would have to tend to the husband. The young woman struck a compromise with the doctor—she would give birth to her child naturally and alone among strangers as long as her husband could be at her side during her labor. It was suggested she read a book written by a man, an expert on natural childbirth, who told her exactly what to expect when she gave birth. The author promised if she learned to breathe properly, the birth would be nearly painless. She liked this idea for she knew she was very afraid of pain and had heard wrenching tales of agonizing childbirth from other women.

Each day she left her small apartment to walk in the park. March brought an early spring even into the heart of the city. Trees along the sidewalks leafed out and in the park flocks of pigeons gathered for crumbs, their iridescent plumage glowing in the sunlight. English sparrows chased each other noisily in and out of flowering shrubs as they paired up to bear young. Along the sparkling river seagulls sailed around and around beneath puffy clouds. The air smelled sweet and damp after the long winter and the young woman breathed deeply. It wouldn't be long now.

Finally one day late in April, the young woman felt a warm flood of water run down her legs. She knew this to be a sign her child would soon be born. Her belly had now grown to an enormously unwieldy size stretching her skin until it shone with curiously translucent striations. Thrown out of balance by all the weight she carried in front of her, she walked to the telephone, taking slow, duck-like, side-to-side steps and called her husband, then her doctor. It was time.

Breathless, her husband arrived home and gathered up the overnight case she'd packed weeks earlier. He called a taxi to take them to the hospital. By now the young woman was becoming afraid. Her belly tightened and she felt a strange pressure, which hurt. With all she'd learned from her books and from her birthing class, she still wasn't sure what would happen next, what it would feel like.

When they arrived at the hospital, a nurse took the young woman away from her husband, "for just a little while." She was told to undress and lie naked on a narrow bed, where the nurse would clean her body and prepare it for birth. Then, wrapped in a white hospital gown, she was wheeled into the labor room where her husband waited for her. He looked anxious. The young woman was very relieved to see him.

By now her labor was in earnest, the contractions bore down on her with inexorable pressure. She groaned as a deep unfathomable pain pierced her belly. Her husband held her hand hard and softly reminded her to breathe as she'd been taught. She wished he would sing her a lullaby with his lovely voice. But she could not ask, she was panting too hard to speak. The pain grew like a mushroom then subsided for a moment before it crescendoed again and again like waves pounding the shore. The young woman begged her husband, then the nurse, then the doctor to please make the pain stop just for a moment so she could rest. It was too late. They could do nothing. Her body felt like a runaway train. There was no stopping this baby bearing down the birth canal and erupting into life. For one fleeting second the young woman wished the natural childbirth expert would burn in hell. Each wave of pain opened her womb a little more, preparing the way for the baby's passage.

Suddenly, a loud noise escaped from her throat, and her body stiffened with a new sensation. With all its might, the baby began pushing its way into the world. Her bed was quickly wheeled into the delivery room. Her husband was left behind and alone to wonder what was happening. "Push, push," coached the doctor and he pushed his large hand on the outside of her belly as if it were a tube of toothpaste. She pushed and strained until warm liquid again flooded between her legs that were strapped wide apart on the birthing table. Dimly aware of the nurse at her head holding her hand, encouraging her and comforting her, the young woman gave one last enormous effort. In that moment, her child, a son, slid out of her womb, wailing and gulping for air—from fish to bird in a second. Exhausted, the young woman watched with tears of joy running down her cheeks as the doctor laid the blood-streaked, naked infant on her empty, flaccid belly. Her child was born. A gift. Her body had conceived this small miracle and cradled his life. For a solitary moment all others around her melted away. The young mother was conscious only of her tiny son—he was of her and she of him and would always be. In that moment she felt a wash of pure love come over her for this little April boy.

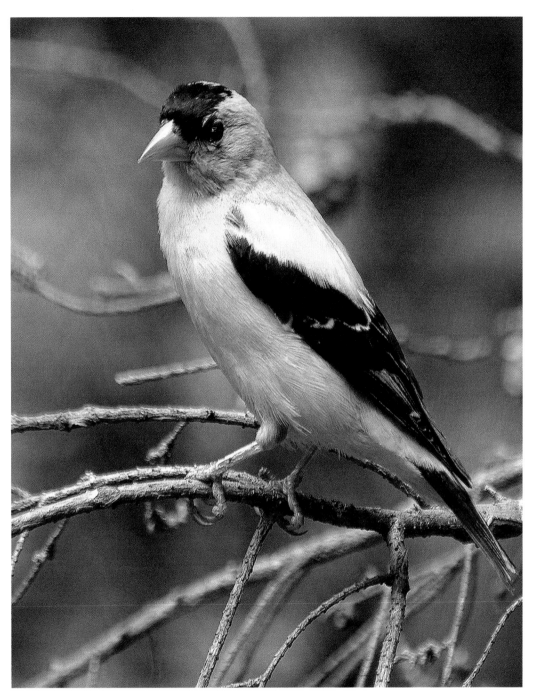

"Yet few think of pure rest or of the healing power of Nature."

_John Muir_

# Old Souls

I come from
a slow-shifting landscape where
worn hills were once dressed in oak and spruce,
where grassy places rolled and welcomed wind.
Now hills thinned of forest sprout dwellings on tarred acres.
I know there are places, which quietly slink back home to a time before.
Here stubborn grasses break cement in abandoned neighborhoods,
juniper and scrub root in idle fields, swamps purple and fill with loosestrife.
I've seen the forest creep across a hill, but to rise long and straight
invites the axe of an insatiable human appetite.
Before me
old souls stepped along my worn woods trail and into
geometric fields, tamed and high with corn, through rocky pastures
bound with venerable walls of stone (built to keep out and to keep in)
past barns, red and redolent of horses, cows, and sheep, home
to historic houses, wrapped with tidy gardens, blue with delphinium
preserved by nostalgia in perpetuity.
Before them,
native people roamed unowned places unfettered by proprietary cravings;
old souls abiding on a wild earth leaving only artifacts for footprints.
And before them,
when giant fingers of ice undressed a wounded landscape,
left scars on fertile, rainbow-colored hills and carved out riverine valleys,
infinitesimal creatures multiplied until the earth settled into its skin;
a forest seeded itself raising spires skyward and filled its dark corners with the breath
of mice and deer, rabbits and wolves; ears rang with psalms of life.
Here, ancients strode home across the mossy trail with backs bent shouldering a good hunt.
One day I, an old soul, will be home
moldering among the ancients,
my bones, historic relics of a time before.

# Legacies

Only in the last year have I come to know and appreciate the legacies written into my family's genetic material. My great-great grandfather's spirit informs mine and I feel I know this man I never met. Louis Agassiz, a nineteenth-century student of natural history and a professor of geology and zoology at Harvard University, founded the Museum of Comparative Zoology in Cambridge, Massachusetts. Agassiz believed a spiritual power informed all creation. He shared his love of the natural world not only with his students, but also with nonacademic audiences who were beguiled by his inspired lectures. He was a man of passion. His biographer Edward Lurie writes, "To Agassiz, the meaning of the creative process was spiritual, and understanding came to him through emotional involvement in intellectual effort. The study of nature was for Agassiz, the study of the universe, and so he thought of himself as mirroring the grandeur of natural history through his perceptions" (p. vii).

Today twenty-first century scientists continue to search for some indication of nature's order and certain it's there, some, like Agassiz, have begun to acknowledge that nature's driving force might, indeed, be the result of divine intelligence. Agassiz' devout faith in the existence of a divine mind, a supreme Creator, underscored his passion for knowing the workings of the natural world, whether he was observing turtle eggs hatching, examining fossil fish, or studying glacial movement. I would now give anything to meet this vital man whose romantic soul was filled with hope, optimism and an undaunted enthusiasm for the world in which he found himself. I feel his curiosity and drive to learn deeply in my bones.

I can only imagine that the seeds of this passion were passed down through his daughter Pauline to his grandson, my grandfather. By all accounts, Louis Agassiz Shaw was a deeply intelligent man. As a boy, he spent much time studying nature, collecting birds and their nests and eggs and cataloguing his specimens much like his grandfather had done years before. But by the time he entered Harvard, his infatuation with nature was spent. His studies suffered from his penchant for carousing until eventually, he dropped out of college.

In his journal, Louis portrays himself as somewhat of a hypochondriacal dilettante without any particular ambition. Family wealth didn't encourage employment. My grandfather languished in boredom and it wasn't until he met and married my grandmother—a beautiful, fiery, aspiring artist—did he find himself once again intrigued by the sciences. I wonder if impending fatherhood and his new role as husband obliged him to take life more seriously and to find something worthwhile to occupy his time.

Louis began his studies in earnest by inviting professors from the Massachusetts Institute of Technology to spend summers at his family's estate in New Hampshire and built a laboratory to lure them into continuing with their own research in exchange for tutoring him in the sciences. These summer sessions finally paid off and L. A. Shaw went on to co-invent the iron lung.

I didn't know this grandfather either, but I have a photograph of him. Surely he bequeathed his everlasting brown hair and the Agassiz hooded eyelids to my mother and me, and like his grandfather before him, his gift to me was an abundant curiosity about the natural world.

My mother, Pauline Agassiz Shaw, was endowed with the gift of her great grandfather's boundless imagination. Her high cheekbones, fine lips and quick laughter, I think, were also gifts from her father and his grandfather. It was she who stimulated my imagination with her love for nature's creatures, all things bright and beautiful, both real and imagined.

My mother loved to write. As a child she wrote and acted in her own plays and later kept volumes of secret journals chronicling her life. She told me she desperately wanted to write her story, but in the end she was too unsure of her voice to pursue this dream. Instead, she expressed herself in her garden, her needlework and the small dioramas she made with perfectly scaled furnishings and little folk brimming with her secret humor. My mother lost herself to brief moments of happiness in these dreamlike rooms even if she wasn't able to give full expression to her passions and creative energy. All the magical creatures that lived in her fantasy and in her beloved world of nature could neither keep her demons at bay nor bring her peace. I always pictured my mother as flying with a single wing. I'm blessed with this rich genetic treasure, blessed to know the lineage from which I've sprung. My spirit is nurtured by the notion that these people still live in my children and me.

# May

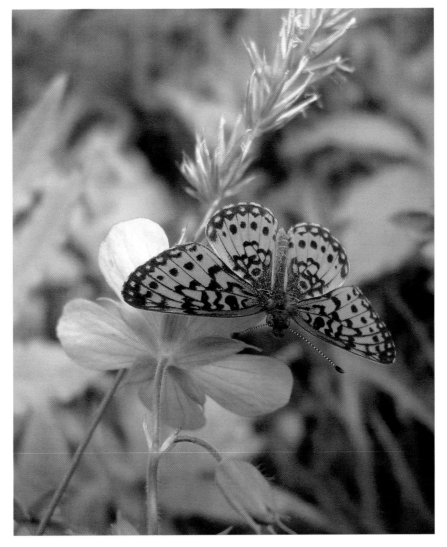

"We are like butterflies who flutter for a
day and think it is forever."

*Carl Sagan*

# May Journal

*May 5*

Today is Rosie's birthday. Born two years ago, she was the last female unspoken for in litter of a dozen golden puppies. On a hot July afternoon a tiny bundle of fur was put in my arms and I was in love the moment Rosie nestled into my neck and licked my nose. Ever since she's been my miracle dog. To celebrate, I bought her a new leash, a collar to match, two chew toys and a bakery cupcake with an elephant frosted on the top. Arriving home with her presents, I toss Rosie a squeaky toy, put a candle in the elephant cupcake and sing "Happy Birthday." She watches me with a mixture of perplexity and eagerness on her face as I divide the cupcake and give her half.

*May 6*

These mornings I'm curious to hear whose voice will sing in the dawn. Lately the cardinal has been the first bird to greet the light with his "cheer-cheer-cheer." Then tucked high in the spruce a robin begins to sing, "cheerily-cheer-up-cheerily." From somewhere inside the viburnum bush a tufted titmouse calls "here, here, here." His mate at the feeder begins to squeak and quiver her wings. And now, closer by my window a cluster of male goldfinches perch in the viburnum's greening branches to preen their new yellow feathers and prattle. They look like miniature daffodils. Listening to these bright salutations, how could I not wake up to celebrate the day?

There's a moment of silence while the sky brightens and I look up through the sky window at the cloudless blue and inhale deeply as if to take this pure blue into my lungs. I feel so alive at this very moment and so grateful not to be as consumed with the dark anxiety that's plagued me the past several springs. Breathing deep breaths I remind myself I'm pulsing with life no less than the small singing creatures outside my windows. Silence is broken by the trill of a house wren, who's just returned for the summer. He sings at the top of his voice from the crabapple, adding his voice to the now swelling chorus for the next hour.

When the sun fills the sky, the birds busy themselves with courting and nest building. The only sound I hear is a small breeze teasing the new maple leaves. Each day birch, oak, maple and dogwood leaves swell in size until in a couple of weeks they'll be large enough to make shade. Rosie and I are startled by a loud thump against the window where I've recently hung another feeding tray, which now swings wildly with the weight of a brazen, sooty, black squirrel who's stuffing his mouth with sunflower seeds. Handsome in his glossy coat, he flicks his bushy tail with an air of cockiness until catching sight of me he leaps to the gutter and away.

Down at the bog a bobolink swoops over the meadow caroling bubbly notes on the wing. The music evokes so much feeling I stop to watch his flight and listen; the song echoes in my memory of a child roaming the meadows on her farm flushing up pairs of yellow-hatted blackbirds and listening to the ardent, clear whistling arias of meadowlarks ringing from every fence post. I haven't heard a lark in many years, but this bobolink will do. I'm glad he's back.

Hiding in a thicket beside a ditch, I can just make out a small brown song sparrow, his head tipped to the sky as he pours out a lilting song for his mate fluttering nearby. A community of sparrows inhabit the fallow meadows; they make their nests in the low, thick shrubbery and scatter with a whoosh of wings when Rosie and I approach. I haven't identified all the different kinds of sparrows yet—there are so many—but I'm working on it.

On the pond two pairs of Canada geese shepherd their newly hatched yellow goslings paddling in tight formation between their parents. These are the first babies I've seen this spring. Breaking rank the goslings drift closer to their mother in a clutch of gold fluff. I imagine the softness of their baby plumage in my fingers. Father goose eyes me, then Rosie. He hisses a warning and firmly steers his family further out in the black water. The two life partners are attentive and vigilant parents even though their babies are capable of feeding themselves.

Rosie and I walk along the far ditch toward home. A green frog peers up through a quilt of emerald duckweed covering the still water. He croaks once, then ducks under the surface when my shadow reaches him before I do, leaving a clear patch of dark water. A cabbage butterfly hovers over a patch of bluets whose hearts are shaped like golden stars and a dozen small silver-bordered fritillaries cluster on tall, yellow mustard flowers growing beside the ditch. The tops of their orange wings are dotted and rimmed in black while their undersides are creamy with silver patches. I've never seen so many at once.

## ~ May 9

The red maple at the end of our driveway is filled with light. The old tree is missing large branches lost to storms and disease over many years and it looks particularly ragged this spring. But today a million clusters of red-winged seeds are ripe and ready to spin off with the slightest breeze. Baby green leaves are rimmed with pink. I'd thought this year we'd have to take down the tree, but it's glowing with so much life, maybe it'll weather a few more seasons. Decorating its remaining scraggly branches like bright flowers is a flock of goldfinches. They're still hanging on the thistle feeders while waiting for wild thistles to bloom with fresh food when they start their families. I'm glad of their company.

Rosie's anxious for our walk and pulls me down the road toward the bog. The shadow of a red-tailed hawk drifts over the cranberry meadow like an errant cloud. At the far end of the pond tiny wild strawberries are in bloom among the blue-eyed grasses that have sprung up along the trail. Bunches of ragged robin have painted the bank of the ditch light pink and follow the trajectory of the sun with a hundred starry faces. Higher on the bank and just coming into bloom, clumps of white daisies bob in the wind and they too flash their canary eyes toward the sun. All along the dry shoulders of the trails yellow and orange hawkweed sway on long stems and show off their bright heads.

Turning into the woods, Rosie and I flinch when a large, fat, black snake slides out of the weeds across our path and into the swamp where a train of painted turtles naps in the sun on a waterlogged branch poking out of the reeds. The forest is redolent with new growth and warm leaf litter. A small breeze sifts through the pines and riffles my hair. Just where the sun's dropped a shaft of light into the forest, a single stalk rises amidst a pair of flat hairy leaves and is crowned with a delicately veined, pink blossom, a single flower shaped like a pouch or a slipper. I'm told lady slippers are colonial wild orchids whose seeds aren't wind-borne or eaten and deposited by animals, but fall beside the parent plant and if the seed can find its way to the soil beneath the leaf litter, it will germinate and send up new leaves the following spring. Lady slippers are shy flowers. Finding the first one in May is a gift not to be taken lightly, because they hide in niches in the shelter of a decaying log in a secluded spot of sun well off the traveled path.

Rosie and I move on down the trail. A single thread of cobweb strung across the way tickles my nose. The path leads through a thicket of high blueberry bushes covered with thousands of tiny, creamy bells. I can almost taste the sweet indigo fruit growing within each flower cluster. Still intoxicated by lovely woodsy fragrances, we leave the forest and walk beside the pond. A dead sunfish lies festering in the sun. Rosie loves its aroma and rolls on the fish until she smells just as putrid as it does. At home I find the most perfumed soap I own and shampoo her until she smells like a gardenia.

I've hung baskets of flowers around the entrance deck leading into the porch. Pink and fuchsia geraniums, sky blue and purple African daisies, lemon yellow dahlias, pink petunias and lavender pansies please the spirit, at least until I forget to water them. In the garden, miniature blue azure butterflies fuss around the pansies. I wish I'd thought to bring my camera. My presence disturbs a robin poking for worms at the edge of the lawn and she flies off squawking an angry rebuke. Amidst a cloud of white blossoms the dogwood is in full and exultant bloom and on the topmost branch a mockingbird pours a repetitive cascade of songs to all who'll listen. The bird watcher's guide says mockingbirds are fiercely protective of their relatively small territories, which they select once in the spring when breeding and again in the fall when they must find a place to keep their winter store of food safe from thieves. It's the male who likes to proclaim dominion over his territory from the highest, most exposed perch he can find. Here he sings an incessant stream of copycat songs—up to six at once. Only late in spring when a prospective mate arrives to settle in his territory, does the male mockingbird sing less as he helps her build a nest.

As I write in this journal, I've consumed an entire bag of delicious cherries with complete satisfaction and a sense of peace after a good day—that is until the feisty red squirrel who inhabits my mind softly chatters and plays with worry thoughts. Will the effort I'm making to deeply examine my life strengthen a growing spiritual foundation or will that foundation be stunted by the persistence of recurrent fears of physical health or concern about the health of my relationships? I counter this squirrelly meddling with the knowledge that maybe I have to learn to live with some fear, which isn't necessarily a bad thing so long as it sharpens my senses and I can balance it with the recognition and appreciation of small delights and unbidden smiles. Less and less do I await an epiphany to shake me into belief and happiness. This is a big change for a woman, who, not so long ago, thought she'd never again feel joy. I comfort myself with the notion that should my world crumble, I've become familiar with an inner resilience I hadn't known was there and which won't abandon me.

## ↪ *May 11*

A dozen little plovers scatter up from the sandy edge of the pond where they've been sunning themselves. They fly over the water in unison flashing their white bellies in the sunlight like a school of airborne minnows. A pair of courting tree swallows executes their own dance in the air with enviable precision—dipping, rising and darting over the cranberry meadow. When the birds tire and fly off Rosie and I walk into the woods, our footsteps muffled by a fresh layer of pine needles. I imagine dozens of pairs of eyes following our progress—raccoons, squirrels, chipmunks, deer, an owl or a fox or a skunk, even a porcupine or a black bear. I know our passage doesn't go unnoticed and I wish I could see behind tree trunks, under leaves, into thickets and between hummocks of grass, but I content myself with the knowledge that Rosie and I aren't alone. Suddenly a noisy blue jay announces our presence and then, with the exception of a warbler's light song, the forest is quiet, but for all the eyes.

The pines and birches are in the midst of letting loose clouds of pollen, which gild puddles of still water and turn my green car yellow. I've never paid much attention to the flowering of trees except for those that shout attention to themselves with their blossoms like crabapple, dogwood and cherry trees. In fact I hadn't realized pines or oaks or maples or birches flowered at all. Their flowers, fruits and seeds, their spring and fall foliage—changes I took for granted. This year I've watched tight buds swell until a leaf or flower opens to the sun. When the flowers have done business with bees and other pollinating insects, their petals curl and fall to the ground and the fruits begin to ripen. When tiny, pale, new leaves mature and grow large enough to make shade and feed the tree, they turn deeper shades of green or mauve.

This spring, all my world seems to be in bloom and all my senses tingle as I begin to see familiar things with new eyes. I'm learning the names of trees, butterflies, birds, insects and flowers just as I did as a child, and sometimes it seems as if I'm looking through those same eyes. My brain and spirit are ascending a steep learning curve, which may never drop off so long as I remain aware and open to all that nature offers me. Learning is unavoidable as Rosie and I walk around the bog, through the woods or into my garden where new sensations, sights and aromas abound and change daily. My connection with nature expands in wonder with each new bit of knowledge. I'm astonished at how much of my natural environment I've taken for granted and now I discover how deep and pleasurable can be a relationship with all living beings as I attend to the minuscule, the larger and infinite progressions of spring's transformations. Poems flirt with my mind and words appear to express my songs. The fifteenth-century Zen poet Basho writes, "It is this poetic spirit that leads one to follow nature and become a friend with things of the seasons. For a person who has the spirit, everything she sees becomes a flower, and everything he imagines turns into the moon." Today is a big "yes!"

Turning into the driveway, I'm overwhelmed by the heady perfume of white and lavender lilac bushes growing in a lanky circle at the side of the house. I keep meaning to prune them severely with the hope they'll thicken and not look so scraggly, but I can't bear to cut the thick old branches. Instead, I clip bouquets of lilacs for the porch until it's filled with the ephemeral perfume that echoes in my memory and must linger there until another spring.

## ⊙ *May 25*

Birds are flying too high across the sky window for me to identify them, but lit by the rising sun they sparkle through the blue air. It seems that the early morning choir singers have stopped serenading except for a few persistent soloists who appear to sing for the joy of it. A mourning dove coos softly somewhere in the cool shadows of the pine and a catbird whines in the viburnum.

On an early morning walk, I find yellow pond lilies in bloom with flowers reaching for the sun, encircled by large, deep green pads floating on the black pond where water striders skate its glassy surface. Beside the trail wild geraniums sport clusters of delicate lavender flowers and are covered with tiny orange fritillaries who've spent the night on their dewy flower stalks and now sleepily open their wings to dry in the sun. Halfway around the meadow wild grape vines climb into the trees by the edge of the path. Their leaves have grown so large they completely hide the tangle of vines where a pair of sparrows hide and warble to each other. Blue toadflax, its tiny bluish lavender flowers atop tall stems, blooms among masses of creeping buttercups hugging the ground with miniature golden blossoms. Turning into the woods where the ground is covered with starflowers, I discover more lady slippers poking out of the pine litter not far from a sunny clearing where sweet fern has leafed out and gives off its musky smell.

## *May 26*

I'm all at once feeling anxious and enervated in anticipation of an annual mammogram scheduled for this afternoon. Every year this appointment is a defining moment for me, after which I'm grateful when another spring passes without a recurrence. How could I not be grateful for seven years of life cancer free? Still, I fear becoming complacent. I've beaten some big odds in this my seventh year since diagnosis; current research tells me my chances for developing a new cancer increases each year not just because I've had breast cancer, but because I'm getting older. The fear is real and most disturbing right now. Only last week a friend told me of a woman who'd died of breast cancer nineteen years after her first diagnosis.

Passing the dreaded mammogram exam after the first year, I was relieved. When five years elapsed without incident, I thought I was home free, but the oncologist said, "Not so fast—give it another five." I'm to think of breast cancer as a chronic, life-threatening illness and this knowledge fuels black moods, which often get the better of me. So I work hard to push away the nagging thought that a cell lurks deep in the recesses of my body, malignant and slowly spreading, hidden for the time being from all my senses and from medical imaging, no matter how sophisticated. Hope and fear coexist and are mixed with a teaspoon of denial, a pinch of panic and an insistent voice commanding me to make my days meaningful. It's hard to tame the eye winking at the future. I don't want today to lose its shine, or its promise to fear. I wonder if I can live in that place between the shore and the sea? With ambiguity, uncertainty and the necessity of giving up control.

Every morning when I wake, I look up through the sky window and watch the clouds. I ground myself by stroking Rosie, who sprawls sleepily beside me. I remind myself I need to know, to acknowledge gratitude for just waking up into all this softness. For the time being I'm done with thinking and get out of bed to go into the garden. A light wind has washed the air clean and the sun is brilliant and warm after days of rain and mist. I'm treated to the dearest sight. Under the grape arbor a chickadee yanks tufts of Patches' fur from an old suet feeder I'd filled with a fistful of her combings after much meowing. I can imagine a tiny nest lined with her silky fur and will remind Patches of her gift to the birds when she complains so pitifully next time I brush her.

I've decided not to replace the perennials, which didn't come up this year because some have transplanted themselves, like the yellow daisies who've traveled a good distance from their original site into odd places in the garden where apparently they'd prefer to be. Rhododendron buds have burst their seams letting loose large clusters of fuchsia blooms. Hordes of bees hum around the shrub and bury themselves in the nectar-filled flowers.

## May 28

The mammogram and ultrasoundings proved negative for any new tumors and the cyst that skulks in my left breast is shrinking. Good. I feel better.

This morning I noticed that of the two pairs of Canada geese raising babies on the bog pond, one has disappeared entirely, babies and all and the second family, a family of four, have only two remaining goslings. What's happening to the geese? Rosie and I walk on toward the upper pond where bursting with unspent energy she leaps into the water for a swim emerging with a guilty grin and smelling like musty bog water. We walk almost daily, but it's not enough for her. Our walks are getting shorter and slower because arthritis pinches my feet and the black flies are out in mass stinging worse than mosquitoes. More and more mosquitoes have hatched out of the still marshy water and can't wait to latch onto a passerby. Walking has become a painful experience lately. Where are all the dragonflies that keep these menaces under control?

An impromptu visit from the Fordyce family gave me the opportunity to look after my grandbaby while her parents sought an ice cream, plant-shopping respite. It's hard to believe she's two months old. She's completely adorable. And now she delights us with big grins. Although her parents dared leave for only a short hour and a half—it was the first time away—I think I passed the "sitter" test and have made myself available for more occasions when the need arises. Even if it doesn't, I want to be with her as much as possible.

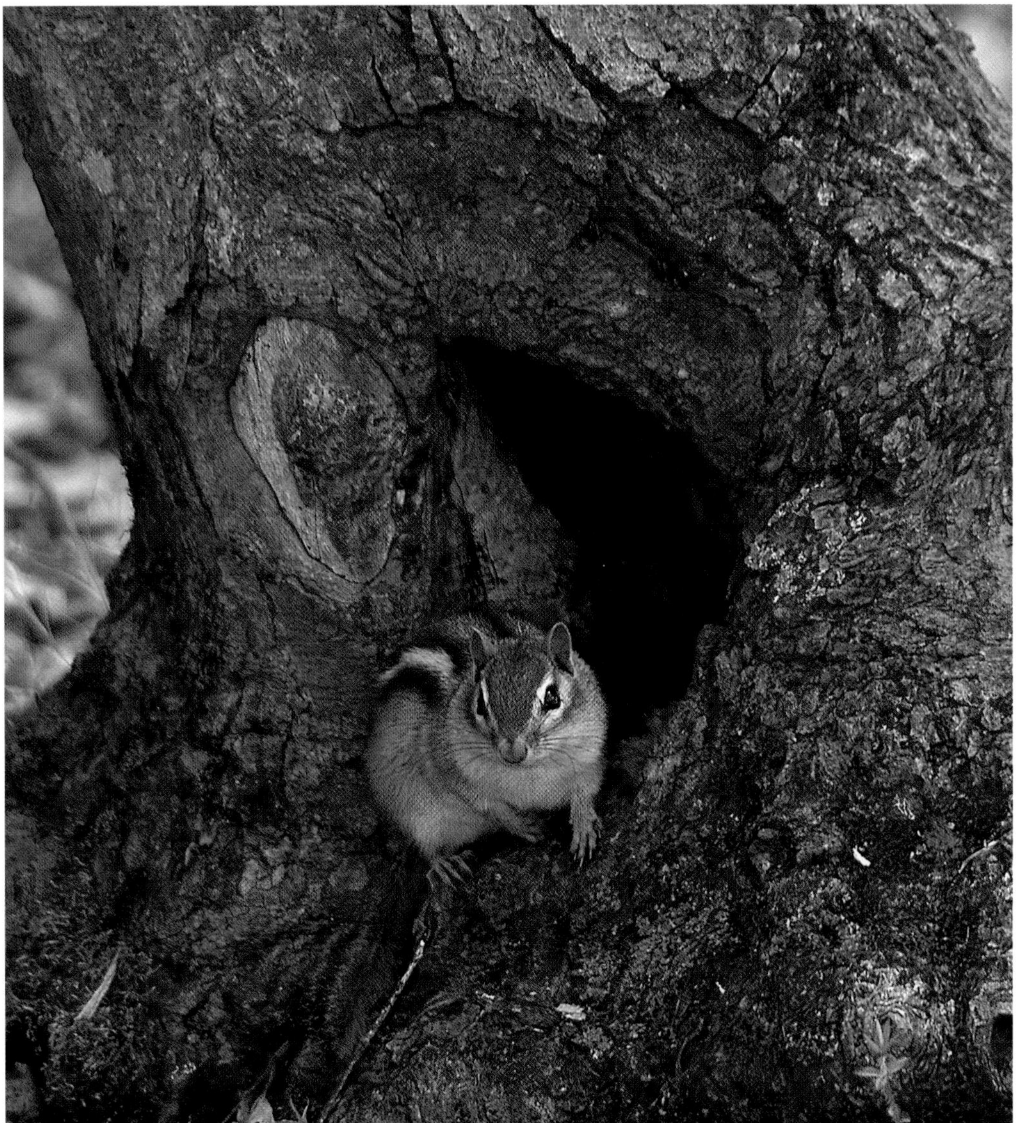

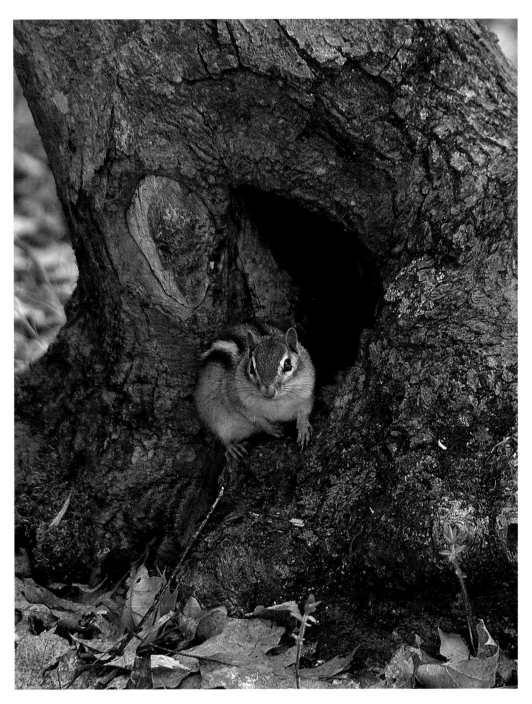

"There are hundreds of ways to kneel and kiss the ground."

*Rumi*

# *I am*

I am bone and boneless
I am flesh and grit I am mind and spirit
I am eyes and insight
I am ears and deaf     I am touched and insensible
I am fruit-filled and fallow
I am shape and slack     I am fragrant and sharp
I am thought and wilderness
I am laughter and lament     I am voice and wordless
I am home and outlander
I am real and reverie     I am rare and ordinary
I am particle and whole
I am kin and solitary     I am you I am me
I am passion and ho-hum
I am unveiled and secret     I am nimble and tedious
I am vulnerable and immune
I am cloud and clay     I am snow and spring melt
I am sunlight and thunder
I am current and swimmer     I am moon and tide bound
I am old and I am not
I am love and aversion     I am reckless and wise
I am realized and undiscovered

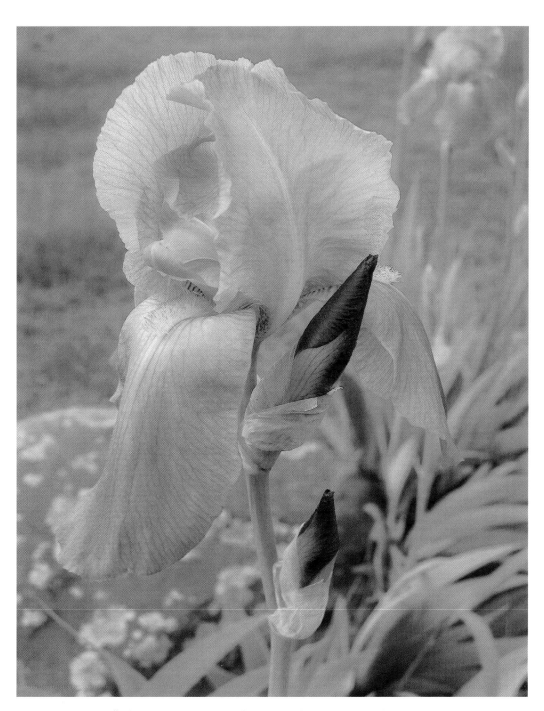

"There is material enough in a single flower for the ornament of a score of cathedrals."

*John Ruskin*

# My House

My house has eyes; north, south, east and west;
never shuttered, draped or shaded, they peek out
on green or bare or white landscapes.
Corralled by gardens, enveloped by trees, I live here
quietly, noisily, happily, sadly, angrily and calmly,
where once there were no doors, where once I went
from room to room on quiet toes, trying different chairs,
where crickets still sing in its dark corners
and mice scrabble through walls and closets
and squirrels invade the attic peak.

In my house paint peels off dingy ceilings and cherished objects
—paintings, signs, my name in antique type, and rows and rows of books
conceal its shabby walls thicker than paint.
Potpourri and flower perfumes mingle
with the fragrance of cats and dogs and us, all pungent and sweet.
The grandfather clock orders time
with a persistent tic-toc, tic-toc, and gallantly tolls the hour.
In my house disorder hides deep in closets, drawers, and relic boxes
brimming with everything impossible to cast away.

But now there's a room overflowing
with sunlight, moonlight, and starlight,
where lilies and violets bloom willingly,
where walls are windows, and a bouquet of found feathers
spray out of an Oriole's nest pinned to a wall
beside an infant's photograph,
where velvet pillows gather on a resting place,
shelves are filled with books and music plays.
In this room in my house,
birds dine and sing by the windows
and the roof is tickled with the scamperings of squirrels.

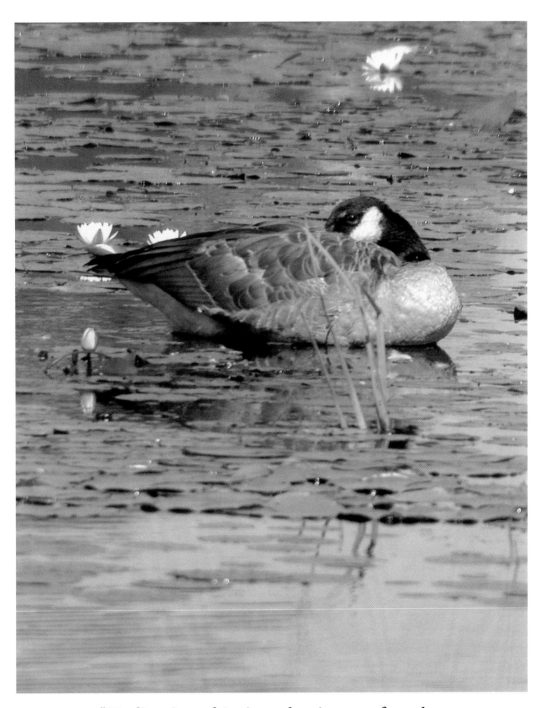

"Healing is embracing what is most feared,
healing is opening what has been closed,
softening what has hardened into
obstruction, healing is learning to trust life."
⁓ *Jeanne Achterberg*

# Coming to Terms

Rummaging through my desk, I've come across a packet of letters my mother wrote to me over thirty years ago. Our last correspondence began when I became a mother. Reading her letters, many in response to mine, has me reflecting what is it about being a mother, a daughter—a relationship so filled with the special intimacy two women can experience and yet so often fraught with complicated and conflicted emotions. At a very early age I was my mother's confidant, a role I found confusing especially when, as often happened, she sensed she'd overstepped an invisible boundary and decided to change from friend into mother. I wasn't ever sure which hat she wore.

Thirty-nine years ago I bore a son, two years later a daughter and eight years after that I became a divorced, single parent. Choices I made to work to make ends meet and later, to finish college so I could find more lucrative employment, were met with family disapproval. My children complained I wasn't like their friends' mothers, but it was my mother who frequently criticized me for not being the mother she thought I should be and for not being there for her. Out of frustration and following marathon phone arguments in which neither of us listened to the other, I began to write my thoughts and feelings in letters filled with hurt and anger and pleading for understanding and acceptance. I was desperate to be heard. As I struggled to carve out a life of my own, to be a mother myself and a wife, my mother and I grew inexorably apart.

As a young adult in the sixties and seventies, immersed in the status quo of the fifties, my world turned upside down in the shadow of enormous changes taking place in our culture—Vietnam, civil rights, women's liberation, the environment, the assassinations of compelling leaders and the shedding of stultifying values and traditions—left me reeling. It was a world alien to my mother, but it was one filled with possibility for me. As the life of predictability I'd come to expect turned upside down and a larger one pressed in on my consciousness, I discovered I had the opportunity to be a different woman from the one my mother and the post-war culture had prepared me to be. But I hadn't a clue where I was going or how I'd get there. Possibility isn't always an easy path to negotiate and in those days I was often afraid, afraid of not being a good-enough mother, of being alone, of not pleasing my family, of not living up to my own expectations and of not knowing where the road led. What was I going to be? The me I'd known for thirty years had become restless and unfamiliar. She let her hair grow, she wore weird clothes, picked up new slang and developed a passion for arguing the issues. Concepts I still valued like kindness, courtesy and accountability appeared to be trashed by the new generation who systematically tossed out the proverbial baby with the bathwater, yet the open raging against injustice and the invitation to be free to be myself appealed to me.

It disturbed my mother that I had feelings and ideas different from hers, and looking back I can see that her disapproval stemmed from her fear of losing me as my exploration of possibility pulled us apart not only philosophically, but in more fundamental ways. Gradually as my world widened and grew beyond hers, I rejected many of the values my mother held dear, values I came to see as superficial and hypocritical. She witnessed me stumble and fall and pick myself up in a clumsy effort to cobble together a life never dreamed possible for a woman of her generation. My life was messy. Her response was inevitably, "I told you so." Or she'd complain and become just plain needy just when I most needed unconditional support. That my mother couldn't let me go, frustrated and angered me and also made me doubt myself.

Rereading my letters to her, I'm struck by the force of my desperate need to justify my worth. I begged for her approval and implored her to allow me to make my own way with her blessing. Today my letters sound insufferably whiny, yet I remember the enormous lengths to which I went to forge a new and viable connection with her. After all, I loved her dearly. Her responses countered with defensiveness and hurt and even on paper she confused her own feelings with mine. But in one unforgettable letter written several months before my mother died, she told me she'd had "a veil" over her heart all her life that prevented her from having the level of empathy she knew I'd craved and she acknowledged she hadn't supported me as I'd needed. Tears of gratitude welled in my eyes for here was the promise of healing I'd wished for. But it was too late. The nascent, deep understanding between us was cut short by her sudden death.

Reading her poignant letter, tears come unbidden and I'm once again making peace with my mother. I understand better now why we had such a difficult time together, especially in her later years when I was afraid she'd die and leave me alone with all of our unresolved business. I let myself think less of my mother convinced, as I was, that too often she gave into her many ailments, some either hypochondriacal or iatrogenically induced. It was impossible for me to accept her woundedness with all my heart. For so long I'd felt obliged to make my mother happy and when I understood it wasn't possible, that it wasn't up to me, I began to recognize it was my desperate need for her approval and her desperate unhappiness that erected a barrier to expressing our deep love for one another. The saddest realization comes now that my mother's not here: She yearned for her own mother's love and appreciation, which was never given, just as I ached for hers, which was conditional. My mother also needed her daughter's approval of her as a mother no less than I needed her acceptance of me as her daughter. Blinded by my own need, and overwhelmed by hers, I didn't give her this gift.

Now thinking about love, betrayal, disappointment, sadness and more love, after years of diligently trying not to become my mother, it's ironic how some of the things I like best about myself are those characteristics that came from her. Her love of nature, of creatures, of flowers and mystical beings, her remarkably keen sense of humor, her laughter, which came from deep in her belly, her generosity, which didn't as I'd always imagined come with strings attached, and her creativity—all of these parts of her are the parts of me I cherish. If I were to write her now, if this were our letter of forgiveness to each other, I'd say, "Wherever you are, Mum, I understand, finally. I miss you and love you."

# June

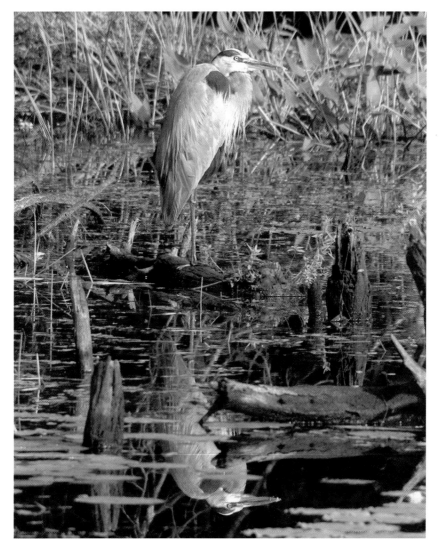

"In wildness is the preservation of the world."

*Henry David Thoreau*

# June Journal

## June 3

An eastern flycatcher yanks a beak full of Patches' fur from the suet feeder hanging in the grape arbor. I've filled it twice this week as a titmouse and more chickadees have come to gather soft combings to line their nests. Patches isn't a happy cat and wails when I comb out her mats, but I try to comfort her by telling her it's for a good cause. She doesn't buy it.

I'm upset to find not one goose family down at the bog today. The two families with their flotilla of gold babies are gone. My spring joy has been to make friends with the goose families.

I've not seen any bobolinks either. The couple I heard a few days ago has disappeared along with the geese. What's happened? I've so loved to hear their songs. How I miss them all. I truly fear the bog is changing too rapidly this year and becoming less and less an inviting habitat for wildlife. I think many creatures are being displaced by the reconditioning of fallow cranberry meadows and by the poisons being used to control insects and weeds. As I make my way around the bog trails my thoughts run from depressed to bleak until they're interrupted momentarily by the sight of a profuse display of ragged robin with masses of pink stars nodding at the sun. They've escaped the mower's blade.

Still the bog's become a wounded place, though perhaps less permanently than the many acres in my neighborhood that sprout trophy houses landscaped with sterile lawns, yards of bark mulch, nursery-grown shrubs and pavement. The few tall pines left stand tall to dry in the hot sun. Today it's as if my body is mirroring my dispirited heart with its stiff, sore joints and the small headache that's nagged me since dawn. A glass of strong iced coffee eases the latter and determination to work a couple of hours in the garden greases my joints making the stiffness bearable.

### June 6

On the way home from town I saw a doe lying in a field of tall timothy grass showing only her head and her large ears backlit by the sun. I stopped the car for a moment to watch her basking in her resting place chewing on sweet grass, then sped home to get my camera. By the time I returned, the deer was gone and although I was disappointed not to have captured the moment on film, seeing her like that was a gift.

### June 9

It's been a lovely cool week with a couple of days of badly needed torrential, all-day rain. Today is full of extravagant sunshine and puffed-up clouds sparkle in the sky. Mornings are still quiet except for the mockingbird, who carries on from daybreak to dusk from the top of anything tall, the tip of a spruce, a chimney or my roof. I sit in my "place" and listen to Andrea Bocelli and Sarah Brightman sing "Time to Say Goodbye." I'm weeping and straining to sing along with them and wonder why it is that music like this always makes me sprout tears. Nowadays I don't really mind unbidden tears, which flow so easily whenever I'm moved by something.

Andrea Bocelli is no longer singing his heartrending arias and my tears have finally dried, so needing something mindless and mundane to occupy myself, I turn to sorting the burgeoning collection of photographs taken this spring. I'm pleased with the results. So many images have been captured just outside my door, in the garden or down at the bog. There was a time I dismissed subjects like bugs as small, insignificant and uninteresting and now they fill me with wonder and fill my photographs—especially, bees, dragonflies, iridescent beetles and butterflies.

### June 10

In the night I awoke to the gentle plink of rain on the window above me and this morning's sky is still filled with clouds promising rain, but none falls. I'm watching a particularly dark cloud approach from the west and wonder if it will save me the effort of watering my flowers. This warm humidity induces sweat, which pours from the roots of my hair, soaking my head and dribbles down my cheeks and into my eyes. My mother used to boast she never sweated and I don't remember anything more that a light film of perspiration above her lips—a trait, sadly, I didn't inherit. So here I am with a body that's never liked temperatures much above sixty-five. I'd hoped age would dry me up a bit, but it hasn't.

The avian chorus has picked up its tempo having been quiet for the past two mornings. Large and menacing crows perch in the tops of the pines investigating my little sanctuary of feeding stations. They're becoming bolder, coming closer and I'm worried they'll scare away the smaller birds. Towhees and chipping sparrows scratch for food among the dry leaf litter at the edge of the woods out back where an oriole sings hidden in the thickening foliage of a maple. I haven't discovered who my mystery bird is yet, but I suspect it's another oriole after glimpsing a flash of orange amongst the maple leaves. I've learned that a single species, robins for instance, will sing a similar song, but each bird may put his own spin on the song, just enough to confuse the human ear. This may be the case with the mystery bird—it's an oriole who doesn't sound like one.

Now the viburnum shrubs in the front of the house are so thick with leaves, there's little possibility of photographing creatures in the bushes until next fall. Daily I'm delighted by the brilliant cardinals who are faithful to their neighborhood restaurant, along with the bluest of blue jays, the soft, mouse-brown doves and the redwings. A pair of chipmunks bicker beneath the feeders out back and wait for the chickadees and one brazen squirrel to knock seeds down to them. I think the little reds have become feistier since winter, if that's possible. They're constantly squabbling and nattering at each other and tearing up one tree trunk and down another, their BB eyes glittering in the sunlight.

When I finally get a chance to walk, Rosie and I head for the bog. A great blue heron fishes in solitude in the wooded corner of the upper bog pond and isn't at all concerned with our approach so intent is he on stalking his prey. Suddenly he thrusts his head into the coppery water, spears a small frog and flips it headfirst down his gullet. Herons like to dine at dawn and at dusk, but this one fishes here all day.

Not far from our pond is a stand of bare trees, which stick up like a handful of pencils from a marsh where a colony of herons has built a rookery with six huge nests. Some of the rough platforms measure four feet across and each is perched precariously in the arms of a dead tree. Migrating north in April, the herons return to the same rookery to begin the process of courting, mating and raising their young. The parents look ungainly as they maneuver around their huge stick nests filled with two or three even more gangly young who will become quite large before they fledge. The family fills the nest in a tangle of long legs, scrawny necks and exquisitely homely faces with oversized beaks—faces only a mother could love. In the past couple of years I've spent time watching the heron families and photographing them. With my camera steadied on a tripod I wait until a parent flies in from a nearby fishing hole to feed her hungry babies who fight greedily for her regurgitated offerings. Once she's delivered the food, she stands regally on the rim of the nest and preens until she tires of her restless offspring and flies off to a chorus of loud squawking.

This spring the rookery is empty, the stick nests have disintegrated and no heron families are in sight. I've thought of all the reasons why they might have abandoned this nesting site, but never did I think I might be part of the problem. Located by the side of a busy road, the heron rookery has, for some time, captivated passers-by, who stop their cars to watch the birds just as I have done. Recently I read an article about herons in a nature magazine and learned that even if humans observe rookeries from a distance, their presence is an intrusion and herons will abandon rookeries they've returned to for years.

Rosie and I continue on our walk and pass the spot where the other day at the edge of the trail a snapping turtle had scratched a hole in the soft dirt to lay her eggs. Today the cavity has been ransacked and the ground is littered with empty eggshells. It's hard to be a turtle when almost anything with paws can dig up your shallow nest. Tree swallows swoop over the bog pond and scoop up tiny insects. Conventional wisdom says when swallows fly low one can expect rain and most of this week's been cool and rainy. The land seems to have satisfied its deep thirst and now looks more greenly lush than ever.

## June 16

Very early this morning a tiny bundle has been delivered into my care for the remainder of the morning. My grandbaby. At two and a half months smiles come frequently and I detect a trace of humor in the upturned corners of her mouth. Ilaria's beginning to murmur small sounds like a bluebird in response to my gurgling at her. I'm studying her as she drinks her mother's milk from a bottle. Her little hands are perfect with long, long, delicate fingers, which grasp and let go of my finger. When her hunger is satisfied her blue eyes droop and fringes of dark lashes rest on her cheeks like whispers. Wee eyebrows, perfect arches, pucker into a quick unconscious frown and flatten out in sleep as her breathing slows. This precious child, a pool of wonderful genes, a creature of possibility and promise, sleeps in my arms, her hand curled into a loose fist tucked against her cheek and I feel blessed.

## June 17

An enormous yawn courses through my body and soul. I desperately need sleep, deep, dark, drifting sleep after staying awake most of the night. It feels as if I'm being forced to learn lessons in human joint anatomy because each one of mine is stiff and sore. It's got to be the humidity. It's 4:30 A.M. The unexpected clear song of a warbler is audible above the hum of the fan. Rosie lies against me and Patches insists on sitting on top of my head. Both these cozy creatures radiate more BTUs than I can bear, but such uncomplicated love is hard to come by and so I stay still and doze off. In a few minutes I'm awakened once more by an early bird singing matins until one by one others join in. A cardinal sings a solo, then a robin chimes in and a titmouse until the chorus swells just as the night sky metamorphoses from charcoal to blue in a matter of an hour. By now grumpiness overtakes my sleepy psyche and one would do well not to mess with me today.

Rosie wants to be let out and carefully, joint by joint, I lift my stiff body out of bed. The hemlocks are silhouetted against the deep indigo and a breeze has quickened to suck the humidity out of the air making it easier to rise from bed once again to let a whining Rosie in. Claiming the sky, the sun pours down its heat from on high. The singing has ended and only chatty squirrels and squeaking chipmunks break the silence. An entire community of creatures has ushered in the morning for me.

Wild gardens are blooming everywhere—along the roadsides, down at the bog—and even my own garden is happily flowering. Orange hawkweed, blue-eyed grass and oxeye daisies sprout out of the roadside detritus and blue-flag irises open their faces to the sun in the wetlands down at the bog where yellow pond lilies and creamy white water lilies crowd the shores of the upper pond. Buttercups, salsify, daisy fleabane, purple cow vetch and all kinds of clover fill the meadows. On one stretch of the trail, about the length of a football field, I count fifteen different species of flowering plants. A multitude of grasses clump along the trail side, their flower heads glistening in the sun. I'm just beginning to learn names like squirrel tail grass, bristly foxtail and timothy grass. The latter I'm familiar with since we grew fields of it on our farm when I was a girl. I've read that timothy grew wild in New Hampshire until it was discovered as a good food grass for livestock. I pull a stem of timothy out of its clump and chew its sweet end. So far the bog grasses and many of its flowers have escaped the mower's blade.

Growing on the most inhospitable sandy trails are common plantains, which were once called "white man's foot" by Native Americans who believed the plant took root wherever a white man set foot, hence its ubiquitous appearance on this well-worn path. According to Lauren Brown, author of *Grasses*, there are true grasses, sedges and rushes. Until now I've not known more than a few obvious species of lawn grass, clovers, rye and other grains and daily the awareness of so many species of wild grasses growing in my neighborhood teases my learning curve, I hardly know where to begin. It's worse than learning the names of trees, warblers and wildflowers.

## June 20

It's late in the morning and the bog is curiously silent. In the bright sun and dry air, Rosie and I happily make our rounds. Now and again a song sparrow calls for his brown mate hidden in a clump of brown underbrush. Three silent crows take to the air at our approach. There have been no geese on the ponds for weeks and only a lone mallard preens in the sun near the meadow. Usually the tall grasses sing with crickets and other buzzy insects. Perhaps everyone has taken cover from the hot breeze that makes the leaves of the swamp maples, sassafras and wild cherry flutter and turn silvery. Or maybe it's siesta time when most creatures stay out of the noonday sun. Suddenly Rosie and I startle a bobolink, who explodes up from the bank of the pond and bursts into his lilting, hollow song on the wing—a song that breaks my heart, but today I'm overjoyed hearing it and seeing the bird.

### *June 24*

For the past hour I've been watching my little granddaughter sleep on the porch bed, enchanted by the soft sucking noises she makes and fleeting smiles and frowns that pass over her tiny face. What must she be dreaming? It's time to feed Ilaria, but she's sleeping so soundly, it seems a shame to wake her. I'd best call her mum.

The little one has gone home now and I'm meddling in the window box. A hummingbird whizzes in to check out the nectar feeder I've fixed to the porch window with a suction cup. Seeing me, he zips away. Still, I'm hopeful he'll come back now that he knows where the food is. Our walk is delayed until this evening when it's cooler and Barry comes home. I've had a peaceful, completely satisfying day just being with my dear grandbaby.

### *June 25*

This morning I woke up feeling sore and creaky and just plain awful. It's unbearably hot and humid. The sky is thick with clouds so full of moisture; raindrops seem to ooze down in an intermittent sprinkle rather than in a steady downpour. Only when a thunderstorm quickly passes by does the rain fall hard. I've managed to do some cleaning and rearranging of the kitchen, which has temporarily made me feel a little better.

When it clears, Rosie and I trudge to the bog where I see the mower has scraped the banks of the dikes and all the trail sides clean. In spite of this apparent wasteland low growing cinquefoil blooms and tiny shoots are reappearing. I think these wild gardens won't be controlled and I cheer for nature's persistence.

### *June 30*

Finally the air is clean, dry and wonderfully cool. The sky holds a fleet of giant cumulus clouds sailing before the wind. In the garden a pair of pale, yellow cabbage butterflies flutters and dances high into the bowl of the sky until they're lost in the impossible blue. Dragonflies, regular visitors to my garden, pose on the tips of daylily buds where they linger for a while before zipping off. I can't imagine what they're doing—perhaps taking a moment for quiet meditation in their whizzing day. The hummingbird has returned and seems to like the sugar water I've put out for him. Funny, in the shade his ruby throat is dull and colorless.

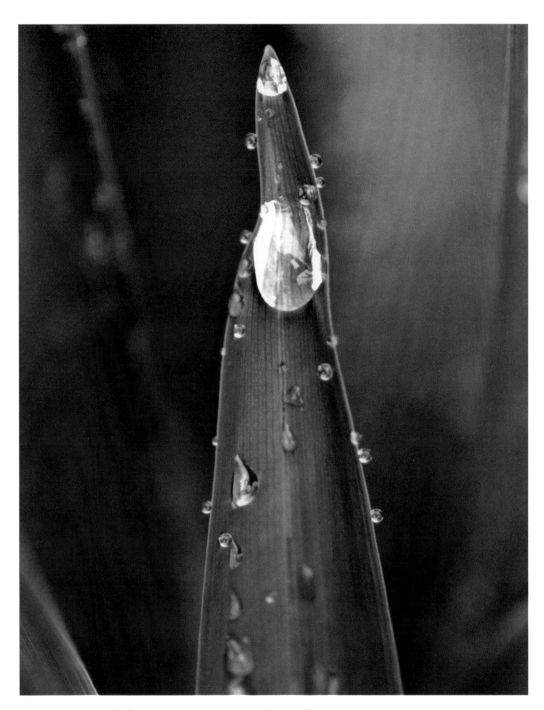

"The moment one gives close attention to anything, even a blade of grass, it becomes a mysterious, awesome, indescribably magnificent world in itself."

*Henry Miller*

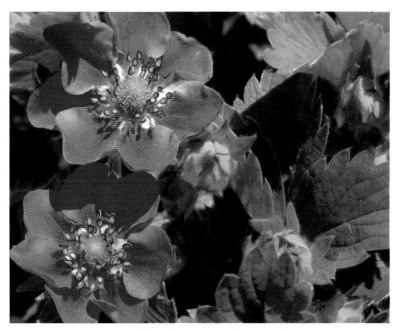

## My Mother's Garden of Roses

She fussed; she pruned and fed her roses,
she coaxed them into flawless bloom, enduring
thorn-bites, plagues of beetles and droughts.

One day I heard her say, "I can't bear it!"
Her cry flew into the endless blue air.
Scarlet-petaled cups brimmed with tears.

"I have a veil across my heart," she wept.

Trapped in the fist of a bud, tormented by beetles,
she fidgeted with one more impossible rose,
forgetting how it loved her back.

In a swift and silken moment her garden
grew brambly, abandoned to wanton blossoms
so red, so golden—too wild to bear.

Her sparkling petals curled at their edges,
and fell petal by petal in a glorious heap
where once her roses grew.

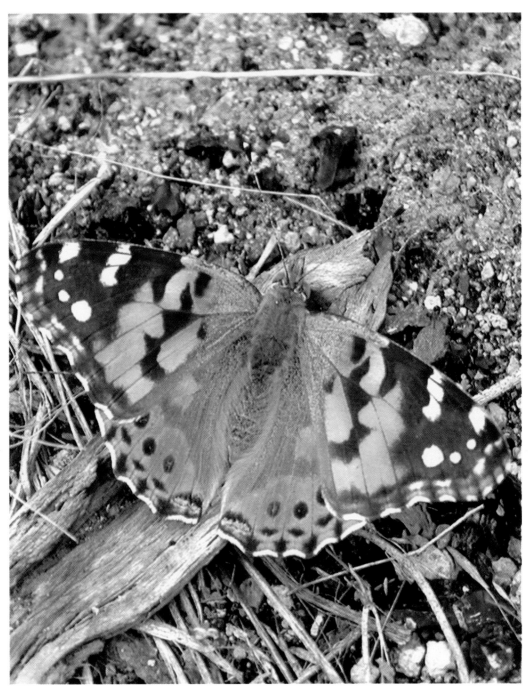

"Like the sky, heaven begins at one's feet.
Look down."

‿ *Diane Ackerman*

# Gardens

"Bread feeds the body indeed, but
flowers feed also the soul."

*The Koran*

I was a small girl of five squatting next to my mother in the garden while she picked beetles out of rose blossoms. Bounded by a low evergreen hedge, this square pocket of silky pastel-colored flowers filled the air with attar of roses and magic. My mother flicked the bugs into a mason jar of kerosene, her lips pursed in disgust. Once she showed me how to pinch a beetle before it chewed a great hole in a rosebud. The nasty greenish-gray insects clasped my fingers with sticky feet as I shook them into the kerosene with the same mixture of disgust and gleeful satisfaction I'd seen on my mother's face.

She told me each rosebush had a name: Marquise Bocella bloomed all summer long, it's sweet, heavy double-pink blossoms glittering in the sunlight; Cecile Brunner bloomed in a froth of pink clusters; Louis Odier bowed to the ground with the weight of its dark salmon blooms and heavy perfume. My mother carefully laid roses she'd clipped to bring into the house in a wide basket she'd set beside us. All summer long our rooms overflowed with vases of fragrant roses, peonies or spring lilacs. I remember how my nostrils tickled with the heady perfume as I sat next to my mother and watched her tend her roses and talk about stuff.

This is what she told me: If you take very good care of a rosebush, it will live for years and years, but you have to keep the bugs off in the summer and feed it with special powder. In the fall you must carefully prune each plant and mound it with straw to protect it from ice and snow. In spring, rake the mulch away so the rosebush can breathe. Sometimes you'll uncover a brown thorny plant that has succumbed to the cold in spite of your ministrations and that can't be helped.

Three wide stone steps led out of the rose garden onto a flagstone terrace bordered by more gardens thickly planted with lush, spiky, blue, delphinium, top-heavy peonies with creamy white blossoms threaded with scarlet, whose heads lolled drunkenly after it rained. My mother told me the tiny ants crawling all over the peony buds were good bugs because they ate the aphids who'd otherwise suck the life out of the flower until it shriveled up and died. I never did see an aphid, but I knew it must be an awful creature if it could do that. As ever, I took my mother's words as gospel—hyperbole and all. In the dappled shade of tall peony plants, miniature Johnny-jump-ups sprouted deep purple and yellow faces. Clumps of red and yellow tulips opened their cups to the sun down at the edge of the apple orchard where hundreds of daffodils bloomed in the spring when the trees were covered with clouds of pink and white flowers and hummed with bees. I liked to sit under an apple tree and listen to the insistent drone of the bees as they drank nectar and watch creamy petals drift down around me like snow.

One year my mother had a vegetable garden plowed out past the clothesline at the edge of the pasture. She raked the earth smooth and marked perfect, long, straight rows with twine before planting peas, corn, tomatoes, beans, lettuce, radishes, onions and squashes. Unable to tend this enormous project by herself, she hired an old man with a disgusting drip always hanging from his nose. He thinned and weeded and watered the vegetable garden and my mother proudly harvested her crops when they came into season, filling her basket with radishes and carrots and beets, which we ate all summer long and into the winter.

I can picture her with her face shaded by a wide-brimmed straw hat, eyes hidden behind Hollywood-style sunglasses, wearing a wraparound skirt that parted easily with an errant breeze to reveal her ivory silk slip and white skinny legs of which she was inordinately proud. It was a feature her three daughters would share—forever-shapely legs no matter their girth size. In the fall, beans and tomatoes were canned and potatoes, onions and squashes were piled into a dark, spidery root cellar under the garage.

My mother's imagination filled my own with a secret garden massed with flowers where tiny winged creatures sang and danced beneath blossoms. She read me stories from Thornton Burgess and Beatrix Potter books about "Old Mother Nature," "Peter Rabbit," and "Reddy the Fox"—stories that made the meadows and woodlands come alive for me. Everywhere I wandered I'd be on the lookout for Peter Rabbit and his friends.

When I was older, I was given a small plot of earth where a tiny, abandoned chicken coop stood. Here I made my own garden. This half-acre was home to a sheep named Petunia who'd given birth to twins late in the winter and a pair of mean-spirited Muscovy geese who nipped at my legs whenever they had a mind to. I had to cross a pasture full of mischievous heifers who, if they discovered me, chased me right up to my garden gate.

I spent days cleaning out the coop, whitewashed its walls and made gunnysack curtains for its single window. I filled rough wood shelves with Golden Nature Guides and a spiral notebook for making lists of all the things I observed. An orange crate serving as a table and two stools completed the decor. With considerable help, I put up and painted a picket fence around the playhouse and dug a tiny vegetable garden in which I planted radishes, lettuce, carrots and onions. The onions smelled wonderful, as their long green stems grew taller and taller, and I'd eat them raw. Around the perimeter of the fence I planted daffodils and later zinnia seeds.

By the time my mother turned fifty, she'd lost interest in working the soil and harvesting vegetables. Now her gardens were planted with masses of perennials along the border of her yard and were tended by a gardener. It wasn't long before even these gardens shrank and turned half wild. Her fingers had become painfully gnarled with arthritis (when I look at my hands today, I see hers). Yet her eye for beauty never deserted her. At teatime sitting in her special chair by the living room fireplace, she designed and meticulously stitched roses, violets and daisies into needlepoint gardens. From her bedroom window my mother had a view of our old farm and she sewed this pastoral landscape with red barns and a field of cows. Sometimes rabbits, kittens and other small creatures found their way into her tapestries.

Often frustrated by the tediousness of her work my mother would complain that she'd "never finish this" and hold it up for her daughters' approval. Nearing completion of a piece she'd become increasingly fed up and say, "That's it! I've had enough of this. I can't bear to do any more of this God-awful background!" At this point she hired a local seamstress to finish the canvas. I sympathized with her impatience, not liking tedium myself. As young adults, my sister and I often visited our mother for tea, driven by our need to feel the continuity and warmth of her fire as much as for her own need to have her family close by.

The garden that grew in my mother's imagination, the one filled with beauty, lovely combinations of color and a deep love of small creatures, also had its dark, sinister corners where lived fear and anxiety cultivated in her childhood, which took root in her soul tormenting her like ominous, black flowers or chewing rose beetles. As my mother grew older, her fears grew more abundant. She worried about dying, flying, going "berserk," letting go of rage, being dependent and finally the most insidious flower of all, the fear of not being real. Just after she died, I found a journal entry that read: "At this moment I'm feeling an overwhelming sense of unreality. I'm filled with doubt, yet I'm not without some ego. I go from feeling utterly helpless and at the mercy of a panic to thinking I can tolerate it on my own somehow. When I feel I can almost bear the fear, I don't feel so much like I'll go berserk...."

These days my mother's peonies fill my garden with lavish blooms. Their creamy double blossoms bow to the earth with morning dew and tiny black ants cruise tight-fisted buds looking for aphids. One lone lupine survives the winters and sends up its sky-blue clusters in late spring. Bunches of daylilies bloom against the lattice fence along with mounds of coral bells. Much like her garden, mine is stuffed with flowers. There isn't a bare spot of soil. And like my mother, I've fancied an instant riot of color and the look of a mature garden. After years of weeding, watering, deadheading and culling plants that couldn't stand up to my rigorous conditions, my garden finally looks like my fantasy. And like my mother, black flowers sprout in my spirit now and again, but their blooms are short-lived and they don't overspread my soul as they did hers.

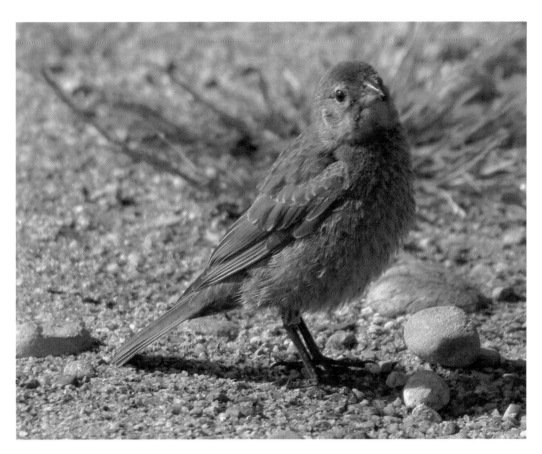

## *When I Don't Feel So Much Me*

When I don't feel so much me
but a fragment of every ephemeral,
flowering, singing thing, I mourn
less things that pass
knowing
such certainty
such finality demands
I embrace all
that's fleeting,
even me.
Still
fear heckles
my heart's song, threatens faith
in ever
lasting.

# July

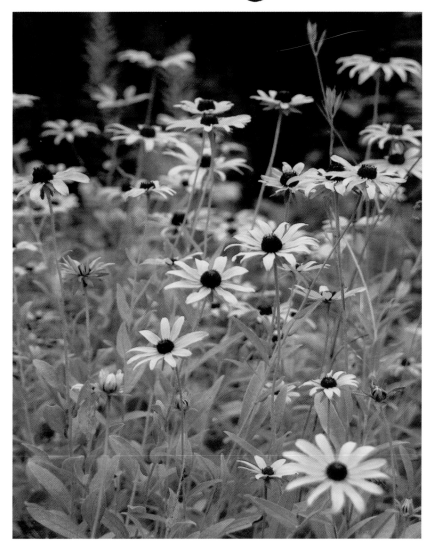

"To those who have not yet learned the
secret of true happiness, begin now to
study the little things in your dooryard."

*George Washington Carver*

# July Journal

### ◌ *July 4*

The sky just begins to turn china blue when a titmouse calls matins outside my window. The air is still and I lie in bed ruminating about living. Until recent years, if I thought about death at all, I was convinced I'd live to a ripe age, or in any case, it would be a good while before I had to confront my demise. So squeamish about the subject and filled with magical thinking was I that when driving by a cemetery I assured my longevity by holding my breath so as not to inhale the exhalations of buried spirits, so I wouldn't catch my death. Cancer vanquished my sense of invulnerability and its attendant denial and now I walk in a lovely cemetery called Sleepy Hollow, breathing deeply and giggling as I think of that old superstitious self.

The heat and humidity have been oppressive these past few days. Arthritis waxes and wanes: One day I feel nimble and the next, every joint screams. This morning after listening to the titmouse and finished with ruminations, I went into the garden to deadhead the daylilies and savor an hour of cool air until the sun beat wickedly down on me. I'm drenched and scarlet with the heat. Walking is a chore and so I skip the daily walk or walk too slowly to call it exercise, which I sorely need to curb the pounds taxing my joints. On top of this I have no desire to curb my appetites. I love food.

Barry and I are taking a very slow walk with the dogs this afternoon. The air down at the bog is thick with moisture. The banks of the ditches are completely shorn again of all that sprouts, buds or flowers. I'm sad and want to go home. The little birds are quiet and even the crows have hidden away in the shadows of the woods. At home I settle in front of a fan set on the porch and watch the hummingbird zip to the window to drink sugar water from the bottle fastened there. She comes early every morning and again late in the afternoon, lingering a few moments before whizzing away.

## *July 5*

Swollen clouds hang like white laundry in a line along the horizon in a sky blue as an iris. It's cooler and drier today and I feel clean and wonderful. Sitting at my desk paying bills, I happen to look out the window and see the rose-breasted grosbeak has come back and is perched on the feeder staring at me. He eyes me for some time before filling his fat beak with seeds and flying off.

## *July 11*

Today I'm in good spirits, having discovered an over-the-counter medication that's relieved arthritis pain completely. Walking is no longer painful and I feel light as air and ready to dance.

Still in my nightgown, I'm overcome with an uncontrollable urge to meddle in the garden. It's time to see who's grown taller, whose buds are swelling and who's blossomed. With feet soaked in cool morning dew, I make the rounds, noticing a pocket of weeds here, a spent blossom needing plucking there. The grape vine has sent its tendrils helter-skelter like a wild Medusa and is in need of severe trimming. Grateful for last night's coolness lingering into this early morning, I pluck and pull and trim, working for a while without being devoured by mosquitoes or cooked by the sun, which is quietly making its inexorable trajectory across my garden. I work until sweat drips off my scalp and into my eyes, until I have to swipe the salty mess with a dirty hand. My white nightgown has become grimier by the moment. In the sun's glow, the garden has come alive. Dragonflies zip by my head. One alights on my shoulder, looks me in the eye and zips away. Painted ladies flutter from daylily to sunflower and pollen-dusted bees make the air hum as they dig deep into flowers. Quickly I go inside for my camera.

Daylilies, scarlet bee balm, a rainbow of zinnias, golden yarrow and blue bachelor buttons and fuchsia butterfly bushes all tempt a myriad of pollinators. All I have to do is wait until one settles on a flower to capture it on film. Circling the garden I follow a delicate blue dragonfly who zooms from one lily bud to another until he finally stops to drink from a drop of dew drying on the leaf of a black-eyed Susan. It's not difficult to picture this sparkling dragonfly as a magical creature, a fairy like one of those populating my mother's whimsical imagination. The butterflies aren't cooperating and drift from one flower to another without staying for breakfast. Just as I focus on an elusive tiger swallowtail, it flits away. Soon I'm too hot and damp to pursue any more bugs and return to the house to fling my dirty nightgown into the washing machine and myself into the shower.

## *July 14*

Standing at the screen door, I hear a familiar buzzing. Mrs. Hummingbird is back, but before alighting on the bottle, she hovers in front of me and looks at me for what seems like a long time before she hums to the bottle for a long sip. Then she buzzes over to the petunias growing in the planter box. What a treat!

The garden is looking fine. All the lilies are in bloom and fill the beds with red, salmon, yellow and orange blossoms. Zinnias are showing off their hot primary colors next to the crisp blues of the last year's bachelor buttons, which have reseeded themselves. Cleome, black-eyed Susans and cosmos line the fence. I love the blues of the bachelor buttons, ageratum and salvia
most of all because they cool my spirit in this heat. A grapevine, planted two years ago by a bird, snakes along the garden fence and is filling out with huge leaves, which protect tiny bunches of green grapes and little birds from the sun. Birds have also graciously planted black raspberries at the back of the yard, which are just now ripening. Rosie and I go to pick some. I gather the ones growing high in the brambles and she nibbles at the lower clusters of berries. Their serendipitous existence has made them all the more delicious. I eat until my fingers and tongue are stained deep red.

## July 24

Mrs. Hummingbird is here for breakfast and is a delight to watch especially when the sun lights up her iridescent green back-feathers. Even though she's missing the ruby throat her mate sports, she's lovely nonetheless.

During the past week a small miracle has occurred down at the bog. Where the trail sides were shorn, small ferns and Lilliputian wildflowers have reseeded themselves or have sprung up from buried rootstock. I should have known nature would prevail and heal the scalped places in spite of herbicides, pesticides and a cutter bar. I was there very early this morning to escape the heat and spotted a green heron fishing in a ditch. Compared to the great blue, this bird is small, has short legs, a shorter neck and wears a black cap. His back and wings are gray-green and like his larger cousin his beak is long and sharp.

Beside the trail following the shore of the upper pond where the mower can't reach, a monarch clings to a milkweed blossom and is chased off by a tiger swallowtail. Fluttering its velvety black wings dotted with blue and orange spots a spicebush swallowtail drifts across our path and disappears into the woods. Spangled fritillaries cluster on flowering grasses and a few painted ladies and skippers dance over the near flowerless landscape. I'm treated to a rare butterfly gathering today.

I've begun to look closely at butterfly wings through my camera lens. What I've learned from reading is that butterfly wings are clear as glass with veins webbing through them. They're covered with thousands of overlapping rows of minute scales, which are easily rubbed off when touched even by the air when a butterfly is in flight. I imagine butterfly scales falling into my garden like pollen dust.

When birds nip at a butterfly's back wings, deceived by the false eyes glaring at them, their attacks leave ragged holes, yet the insect still flies in spite of large chunks of missing wing. Now I understand why at summer's end I've seen many dull and tattered butterflies. Monarchs escape avian predation; because they taste so awful, birds vomit. And because a viceroy looks like a monarch, feathered predators avoid them also. In certain species of butterflies the tops of the wings are brighter, while the undersides are drab; this is especially so for the tiny azure blue who communicates with others of its species with its bright open wings and closes them when it wants to blend with its surroundings.

I've often seen butterflies basking in the early morning sun to warm their wings for flying or come upon a couple of male swallowtails puddling in a wet spot of soil, where they drink mineral salts to enhance their virility. I liken these behaviors to my stretching my body parts before rising in the morning and taking my vitamins—although I'm not concerned about virility. While most animals like me can't see ultraviolet colors, butterflies can and this helps them find nectar-producing flowers, which stand out from other vegetation around the bog. Oxeye daisies, Queen Anne's lace and summer asters have been razed along the bog ditches and trail sides, but pockets of loosestrife, joe-pie weed, milkweed and button bushes are letting loose their perfumes into the air to attract what butterflies are left here. I do miss the profusion of flying flowers this summer but am grateful to the ones who've remained.

Of all the airborne insects, dragonflies and damselflies fascinate me the most and both are flourishing around the bog. They come in all sizes and colors, skimming across the water's surface, flitting over the sunburned trails into the woods or down the road to my garden. They're quick as lightning; they can hover, fly sideways and backward, execute aerial acrobatics like mating on the wing and are second to none, except perhaps the hummingbird. Mosquito dinners appease their voracious appetites and this fact alone should confer on dragonflies the status of hero, given the abundance of mosquitoes in my neighborhood who'd otherwise be happy to dine on us.

The bog provides a perfect habitat for dragonflies with its ponds, swamps and woodland. I see Northern blue damselflies with sky-blue bodies and glittery wings, common green darners, calico pennants with spotted wings and large, timid twelve-spotted skimmers who sport distinctive white and black wing bands. There are yellow-legged meadowhawks with red-orange bodies, blue dashers and eastern pondhawks with brilliant green bodies. Whenever I catch sight of one of these magical insects, I think of my mother's fairy clock, the one inhabited by little people with cobwebbed wings who dance inside when the clock chimes.

I've read how dragonflies undergo several transformations during their lifetime, from egg to nymph to adult. Living under water for one to three years the nymph sheds its skin many times. It over-winters deep in the muck of the pond and breathes through gills like a fish. In early summer the nymph crawls up the side of a reed and throws off its last skin to become a gossamer winged terrestrial insect. Amazingly, dragonflies have been around for three hundred million years, long before dinosaurs or birds. Their secret to surviving so long has been their ability to adapt to whatever environment in which they've found themselves.

Native American wisdom tells me that all animals are bearers of healing messages: messages that can heal the body, mind and spirit; messages that remind one to walk softly on the earth and to open one's heart to receive the lessons offered by its creatures. On this leg of my own journey, I've chosen the dragonfly, or perhaps it's chosen me to teach me what I have yet to learn. I've been especially blessed when an intrepid dragonfly lands on my hand and dallies there or when today, a dragonfly hitched a ride on my shoulder as I walked by the pond. Darting before me on delicate wings the dragonfly leads me onto the path of transformation. She holds me accountable to my inner self, helps me find the strength to adapt to change with a modicum of grace and encourages me to live comfortably in my skin as a survivor of breast cancer. Today I want to dance with the dragonfly.

# The Dragonfly

"Today I saw the dragon-fly
Come from the wells where he did lie.
An inner impulse rent the veil
Of his old husk; from head to tail
Came out clear plates of sapphire mail;
He dried his wings: like gauze they grew;
Thro' crofts and pastures wet with dew
A living flash of light he flew."

*Alfred Lord Tennyson (from "The
Two Voices," lines 8–15, 1833)*

In spite of my whining, this summer's weather has been clear and reasonably cool with enough rain to keep some of the vernal pools damp. Just when I worry about a lack of moisture, the sky drops a nightlong rain to soak the earth and plants grow taller before my eyes. I'm convinced plants like sky water better than earth water. A sprinkler doesn't quench the garden's thirst the way the heavens do.

Today the sky is clotted with towers of clouds whose huge white puffs rise into the blue dome, like thunderheads not quite ready to let loose a storm. These formations are incredibly arranged with water drops filling the bottom of the cloud and ice crystals, the upper part. It's only in very unstable atmospheres that cumulonimbus clouds (as these are called) gather into lovely shapes, which are then likely to bring rain or some other form of stormy precipitation. At the moment the sun is partially obscured by a large, ominous cloud pile. A light breeze stirs the maple leaves with a gentle exhalation. My breath stirs as well and I welcome the riffling breeze wondering if I'm breathing in unison with the breath of the earth.

Rosie sniffs at a bug crawling across the trail. Not touching it, she follows it with her nose, head down and ears flopped forward. She's concentrating hard on this little beetle. I think I need to get to that place more often. Help me, Rosie.

## ~ July 26

Rosie and I head to the bog in a soft early morning drizzle. Just before turning onto the path a slender doe steps out of the roadside thicket. My heart stops. I don't often see deer so close. She looks at the two of us, pauses a moment and then crosses the road. Rosie sits calmly by my side with her ears pricked forward. Again my heart lurches when a shy, polka-dotted fawn ventures out of the same thicket, spots its mother and nimbly trots to her side. I hold my breath. Then another fawn steps daintily into the road, in the wake of its sibling, and the family melts into the woods. I'm so moved by this encounter tears sprout in my eyes. All the while, Rosie hasn't made a peep.

When we arrive at the bog pond Canada geese float along the shore. They're back! I'm so glad to see them, I call "hello" and several geese turn to look at me with curiosity, maybe even recognition. I've made a practice of talking with any goose who'll listen and some of these may be familiar with this strange human who sings to them like a fool. Rosie and I move on. In the largest of the irrigation ditches a mallard trails seven dark yellow and black babies in the coppery water. She, too, turns to listen as I compliment her on her sweet brood. Who knows what these creatures make of my chatter—certainly, they're curious. I feel particularly blessed by all I've witnessed this morning.

## ~ July 29

Mrs. Hummingbird brought her mate to the window feeder for breakfast. His squeaky voice is deeper than hers and his wing sounds stronger, yet he's more cautious than she. It looks as if he's mastering his timidity with the tempting promise of sweet water. Mr.'s ruby throat is startling iridescent in the sun. His flat feathers are specially cupped to capture light, but reflect it in only one direction, so the sun must strike the bird's neck at just the right angle. A passing cloud can transform his raiment into an innocuous dull shade. Mrs. has a white throat, which doesn't need the sun to shine.

Lying on my sofa bed, binoculars in hand, I'm spying on a flicker who's preening on the topmost branch of the dead tree across the street. Large birds seem particularly partial to this tree. I feel like a peeping Tom intruding on the flicker's private moment. Imagining myself perched on top of a small world roofed in blue, with meadows and forests and rooftops stretching for miles around, I can't resist the feeling of freedom as I spread a wing to peer for mites, find none, spread the other and know I can fly at any moment if I want to.

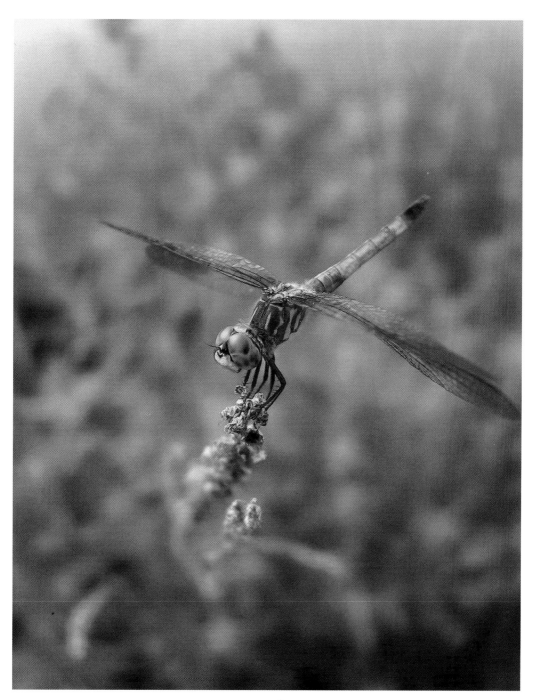

"Every wakeful step, every mindful act is
the direct path to awakening.
Wherever you go, there you are."

*Buddha*

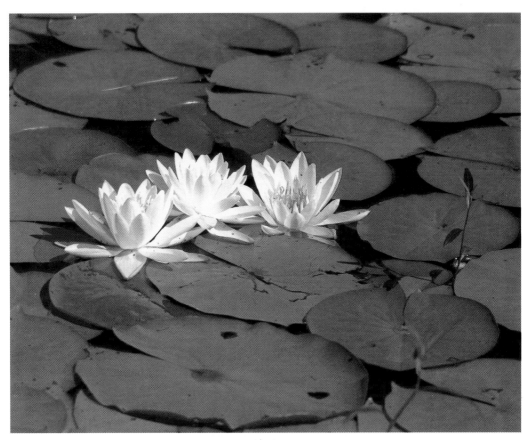

## Water Lilies

Out of the bottom muck they rise on slender stems
like prayers, they slip toward the light
until carpets of lily pads dapple the sun-glossed water.

Leaves, sleek and deeply green, circle a chalice
of ivory blossom holding its cup of sunlight, offering
its gilded stamens to brightly blue and darting damselflies to rest upon.

At dusk, when the bobolink has hushed her carillon song,
when myriads of moon-white petals fold, darkly iridescent
swallows wing low across the starry skin of the pond.

Into the dark blue air, into the salmon clouds
I send a prayer. To fly and swoop like this,
if I could, I'd skim the pond myself.

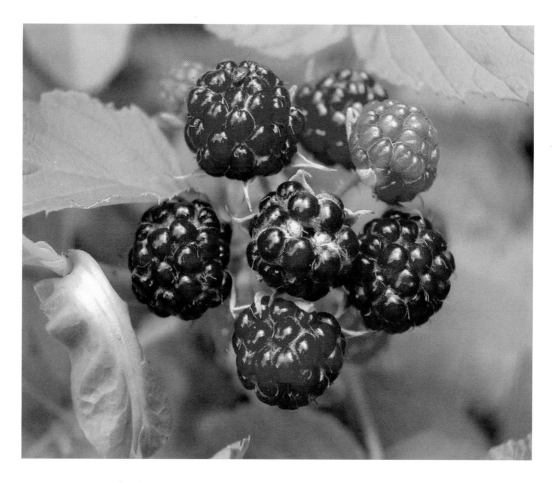

"I do not wonder at a snowflake, a shell, a summer landscape, or the glory of the stars; but at the necessity of beauty under which the universe lies."

*Ralph Waldo Emerson*

# Learning to Observe

Learning to observe with all my senses, to be aware of all that goes on in and around me, is a gift I might never have appreciated had I not listened to the many voices inviting me, even challenging me, to practice rooting myself in the moment. Rosie is my mentor whose lead I follow daily. Wherever we go she sniffs the air and the trail we're walking; she cocks her ears at sounds I can't hear, sees sights I've missed and happily takes in whatever presents itself to her whether it's a beetle, a deer or the scent mark of another animal. Her focused way of looking and listening and feeling is qualitatively different from the ways I've looked at my world in the past. Ralph Waldo Emerson wrote, "To the attentive eye, each moment of the year has its own beauty, and in the same field, it beholds every hour, a picture which was never seen before, and which shall never be seen again." It's true; the same walk around the bog offers new experiences every day throughout the seasons.

Like Rosie, I scan the landscape I'm in, moving from the sky and its cloud formations, soaring hawks and roistering crows, to the bog meadows, its mists of color tinting the trees late in spring and early fall or the snow-blanketed winter meadows; all of it is a feast for the eye. The large sounds of ice singing, pines whistling, oaks and maples swishing their leaves and the lap of water on the bank of the pond and wind; so much wind, gentle, whispering, biting, frigid, noisy and playful wind. How I love the wind! When I've taken in the lay of the land and sky, I focus closer and closer until my eyes come to rest on the ground beneath my feet where I notice small creatures or flowers like ants, a minute flower or a butterfly puddling in the sand. I've honed my peripheral vision to catch quick glimpses of shy creatures out of the corners of my eyes, such as the family of white-tailed deer who last spring slipped silently through the pine woods far off to the side of the trail I was walking. If I'd looked straight at them they would have fled. Some animals don't tolerate direct eye contact and I've learned to give them a sidelong glance.

I scan from side to side when I walk and I look into the treetops in the woods although this habit has led to significant stumbles over roots and stones on the path. Never mind. There are rewards for stumbling, for having to slow down. I also pay attention to the time of day when it's likely I'll see creatures going about their business such as early morning, late afternoon and dusk. Deer come out of hiding to browse the cornfield and there's a burst of activity at the feeders with much twittering before the cardinals, sparrows and nuthatches rise in the morning or return to their roosts for the night. Evening invites nightjars, coyotes, tree frogs, bats and crickets to sing. Raccoons hunt at night and skunks clean up under the bird feeders. By early morning night creatures take shelter in holes and deep in thickets while birds awaken to sing in the first light of day and the squirrels scamper over my roof with cheeks full of seed.

Learning the art of photography has made me particularly aware of light. Not only are animals active in the early and later hours of the day, but also the light at dawn and dusk offers more appealing images than those shot in the harsher, flatter light of midday. I seek out shadows cast by a slanting sun etching the rough bark of a tree, the shadow beneath a toadstool or a dragonfly's wings on a grape leaf—shadows of any kind lend mystery to my images and imagination. I look for the concentrated light on the landscape when the lowering sun tinges everything gold and at daybreak, the soft pink light of early morning or gray mists of a cool dawn. Little by little I've become familiar with birds and their songs, with the names of trees, wildflowers, insects and other fauna. It's a challenge to figure out animal communications, whether they're scratchings in the underbrush, inside my walls or howls and screeches, and rustlings in the dark. I may never know what the coyotes are saying when they yip and howl out in the cornfield, but I sense their community and need to let others know of their presence. Bird language is easier to translate; they call and sing and use body language to communicate with each other—language not so different from ours, such as combative crouching, attacking behaviors, angry chipping or shrieking, or playful chasing and coy avoidance females often engage in when courting. Some birds warble gently to one another and even beak-kiss.

Tracks and other signs of wildlife have become more visible, but I've yet to read the meaning of these signs. Maybe someday when my learning curve isn't so steep I'll practice tracking animals. I do stalk, however, and as I try to blend in with my surroundings I know I must keep downwind of whomever I'm following and I'm less easily seen if I keep the sun behind me and pretend I'm a tree. If I approach a Canada goose and she becomes aware of me, talking softly to her I stop and wait until she continues grazing before moving closer. I don't want to intrude upon her circle of safely, a circle most creatures have to protect them from predators, a circle, which in my own human way, I have too. Learning to observe with "the attentive eye" allows me behold sights that I've "never seen before, and which shall never be seen again." I won't forget these gifts of healing.

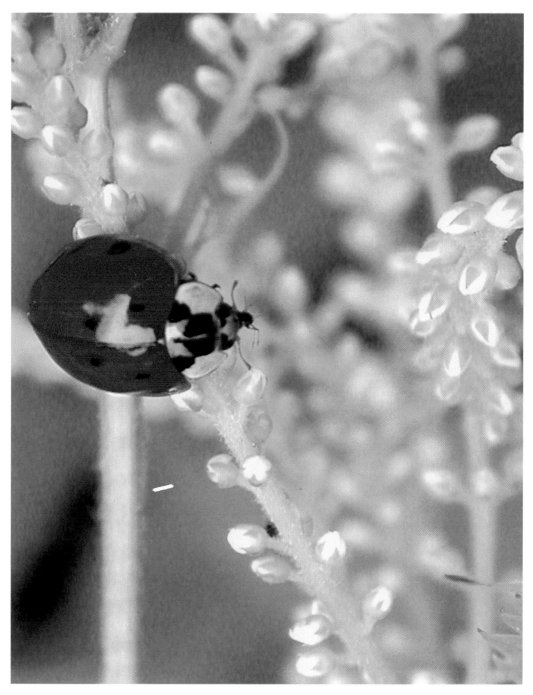

"Come forth into the light of things. Let
nature be your teacher."

⟨~William Wordsworth

## *If You Want To*

If you want a glimpse of eternity, stand on a night hill and see a galaxy of stars.
If you want to see the world go round, watch the moon and stars drift westward.
If you want to feel the earth squirm your toes in mud, tiptoe in mossy places.
To taste the crystal imminence of snow, stick out your tongue in silvery air.
If you want to feel the breath of the earth let the wind touch your face.
To hear the hum of the Universe listen to bees in a June meadow.
If you want to taste an entire season, bite a summer peach.
If you want to taste green nibble tips of timothy grass.

If you want to hear music listen to dawn harmonies, sighing trees and singing frogs.
If you want to see the sun on a dowdy morning look into the face of a sunflower.
If you want to smell the sweetest perfume, sniff lilacs, lilies and milkweed.
If you want to smell green, walk in spring woods or just mown pastures.
To see true artistry watch the sky blush when the sun goes down.
To know courage, find a dandelion poking through cement.
If you want to know the woods walk into it on quiet feet.
To see the bluest blue, look into the sky in May.

If you want to walk on air, drift on silky wings like a butterfly over a field of sunlight.
If you want to see industry, watch a spider spin her lace between two blades of grass.
To know tenacity, watch gray lichens hold fast to granite or mussels cling to a pier.
If you want to fly, let your thoughts take wing with a flight of geese.
If you want to be awed, look an elephant in the eye.
If you want to play float like an otter, roll and dive.
To stop time fish like a great blue heron.

# August

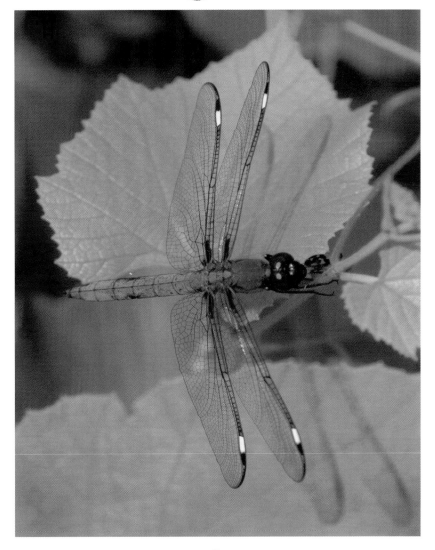

"The dragonfly
can't quite land
on that blade of grass."

    *Basho*

# August Journal

## August 3

How fast time hurtles by! And these days it seems faster than I've ever experienced it in other years, in spite of my efforts to stay focused in the present. It's August already and I'm preparing for an African adventure. Anxiety and downright trepidation has inhibited my writing much about the trip in this journal until now. It's not as if I haven't traveled twice to Africa before, but this time the long journey there is solo. My worry list reads like this: First and most important, will the plane crash? Not an unreasonable concern, since prior to each of the first two trips, a terrible crash has made headlines in the news. Will customs pass my overstuffed duffel without ripping it open for inspection? Will there be electricity to power my hair dryer? I'm usually the only traveler to coif hair that's not drip dry and wear makeup. Will Joy forget to meet me at the Malawi airport? The list goes on and on. I've packed and repacked my luggage countless times, weeding out excesses and deciding which necessities I must have to comply with the parsimonious weight restriction of twenty-six pounds. My heavy camera gear takes up most of the weight, which means I'm taking precious few clothes and none of the "necessities" I'd normally pack.

Sometimes I wonder why I subject myself to anxiety-provoking situations like this, knowing I'm prone to worry. Then I realize that once in a while my spirit requires shaking up to challenge its fondness for security and while mindful walking keeps me from falling into the dulling sense of daily sameness, I need to remind myself I can survive fear itself. God knows I'd sooner be challenged by an adventure other than ill health. The fact is that once I arrive at my destination, anxiety falls away like a heavy old coat and I'm eager for the adventure to unfold. An element of danger attaches itself to all my journeys no matter what the destination, whether it's Africa, beating cancer or controlling my habits and learning new ways to be. The process is difficult and filled with trepidation, but happily, arrival at the destination often culminates with the gift of knowledge.

It's rained for days and I take walks between showers, but I'm spared the twice-a-day watering of container flowers on the deck. The ruby-throated couple appears daily to sip nectar. What pleasure they bring me. Mrs. is a funny little one. Whenever she spies me spying on her through the window, she hovers in front of me then whizzes into the viburnum. In a flash she's back at the feeder. We've encountered one another like this on several occasions. I know my presence interrupts her dinner, but for a split second I feel as if a small wordless communication has occurred. When I move away from the window and look out again, Mrs. Hummingbird has returned with her mate and a girlfriend. He announces his presence with loud wing buzzing and the feisty ladies compete to see who'll have first dibs at the nectar bottle. Then all three whir into the depths of the spruce and disappear.

## August 11

These summer days droop with moisture. Down at the bog, tree swallows have stopped their insect-scooping flights over the pond. Canada geese visit now and again but seem to have found more hospitable places to hang out, although it may be they're laying low unable to fly while molting. I truly miss the rafts of geese drifting on the pond. Last August's drought brought weeks upon rainless weeks, which dulled the landscape and left plants limp with thirst. This year there's a drought of wild creatures and the landscape is lushly green, even mildewed in shady places. The cranberries are ripening in the meadow and one fallow meadow, still untouched, rings with exuberant sparrow songs. White-throated sparrows, song sparrows and swamp sparrows pour their lilting songs into the still air while clinging to a reed stalk or hiding in the grasses that escaped the mower's blade. More and more wildflowers have sprung up in the shaved places. Walking home I notice that the cow corn in neighboring fields has grown so tall the stalks pierce the clouds with spiky leaves and millions of pale green husks have fattened until their tassels appear ready to burst into pale yellow and light mauve switches. Heat bugs (cicadas) slice the dense heat with their electric humming celebrating the hottest of days. Just listening to their high-pitched whine makes the heat feel extreme.

At home the garden is busy with birds. The redwings have departed the bog, but a few remain in my neighborhood and bring their young to dine at my house. Cardinals have found their voices once again and call to one another from inside the hemlock. Squabbling house sparrows explode out of the viburnum when Rosie and I approach the house. It's the goldfinches, bright as sunshine, who are the busiest these days while they await the blossoming of thistles and look for mates. Little blue jays shiny with new sky-blue feathers flutter their wings and open their baby mouths to beg for food in hopes their parents will indulge them. The parents ignore the squawking. Chickadee babies and titmice babies follow their parents, who show them how to crack open sunflower seeds. Except for the goldfinches, the adult birds are in the midst of molting and look scruffy in their dull and ruffled plumage.

## August 13

Things I need to remember: I'm a woman on borrowed time, I'm resilient, I can laugh and I'll live one year at a time and be thrilled that I've come through another no matter what it brings. I need to remember I'm blessed with good health, family, the dearest granddaughter and good friends. I'm surviving. No. I'm doing more than merely surviving, I'm living, if not with certainty about the future. I'm left with a niggling question though. Am I giving enough? Sometimes I think I might be doing more giving of myself. I read about "being of service" to a larger world, to the environment, but my ways of "giving back" seem small by comparison with those who dedicate their lives to service. I'm not sure what fits me or what I can be satisfied with. I do know I try to give myself to all my relationships, both personal and professional, in small consistent and connecting ways. Once in a while an illuminated moment occurs when I've connected deeply with a friend, a client, a creature in a way that takes me so completely outside myself; it's allowed something extraordinary to be exchanged. Careful observation during my walks into nature has honed my awareness of what's around me, not only at the bog, but in all areas of my life. Slowly, often sporadically, I've become increasingly attuned to a door opening to a present blessed with more meaning than I'd realized and to a future, holding more hope than not. Such thoughts on the eve of my departure, fitting, I suppose, given my week-long angst over losing control. The danger I feel when embarking on change or an adventure is about losing control. Well, of course. Isn't this the nugget imbedded in all my journeys?

A daydream: I'm careening into billowing clouds, slicing through skies blue as cornflowers looking down at another self walking bound to the earth on the bog trail and feeling as if I'll never see it all again. Not in the same way at least. The flying me pierces the cottony clouds like the cornstalks do and soars on a westerly wind into the forever blue until I land safely far away from home.

Surprisingly I woke this morning after a full eight hours of sleep and I felt peaceful for the first time in weeks. I'm reading Thich Nhat Hanh and the writing of this Buddhist monk comforts me. He inspires me to stay mindful. In his book *Living Buddha, Living Christ,* this gentle man writes,

> Mindfulness is the key. When you become aware of something, you begin to have enlightenment. When you are drinking a glass of water deeply with your whole being, enlightenment is there in its initial form....When you look at the blue sky and are aware of it, the sky becomes real, and you become real. That is enlightenment....To go back to yourself and dwell in mindfulness is the best practice in difficult moments. Mindfulness breathing is your island, where you can be safe and happy, knowing that

whatever happens, you are doing your best thing....You only need to dwell deeply in the present moment (p.117).

And it's true. When I slip out of the present and rush into the future as I've been doing recently, I'm overcome with worry—not so much despair, but worry about finding enough meaning to sustain me when the going gets rough should the plane crash or I experience another kind of crash. I'm not yet confident my amateur practice of mindfulness is up to the task, but I try to reframe worrisome thoughts and to practice recognizing small encounters, no matter how mundane, which bring me joy. I try especially hard to "dwell deeply in the present moment."

## August 16

The morning thundered in with torrential pockets of rain. Leaves and blossoms droop under the weight of so much water. Undaunted by the rain, Mrs. Hummingbird gives in to her hunger and comes to the feeder with her mate and the girlfriend. I'd like to set up my camera to capture them on film but resist the temptation because my gear is packed away just so and I dare not mess with it. No matter, I'm content to watch the birds. The day after tomorrow I fly east into moonrise.

## August 18

The alarm jars me out of a sound sleep early this morning. Rosie knows something is up and follows me from room to room giving me baleful looks. I'm close to tears at the thought of leaving her, knowing I'll miss her terribly. I also know Barry will take special care of her and she'll be fine. But will I? Packs of clouds laze around in the deep blue sky. An eastern flycatcher flaps across our trail with a beak full of dragonfly as Rosie and I make our last walk around the bog for a few weeks. Out beyond the mats of water lilies some geese float silently. The bog is quiet.

Barry drives me to the airport in the afternoon and without fanfare or incident I wave goodbye and board my flight. I have ample time to settle into my cramped window seat, which has less leg room than recent advertisements promised. Economy class is still a lousy ride. With my small carry-on camera bag safely stashed under the seat and my knees touching the back of the seat in front of me, the pilot's voice, with just the right touch of gravel, announces there's a "computer down" and he'd appreciate our continued patience while a part is to be flown up from New York City. Now I'm less than confident of a safe arrival in London. It'll be two more hours before departure and another oozy message from the pilot invites passengers to disembark if they wish. I don't feel like lugging my stuff off the plane.

Hallelujah! The computer is fixed and people are reboarding the plane, that is, all but my seatmate who'd left earlier. Having been paged several times, he's nowhere to be found. In a somewhat less soothing voice the pilot tells us to expect another delay while the missing passenger's luggage is unloaded. A large groan fills the plane. Then a young man jogs down the aisle and takes his seat beside me bowing to the applause of the entire cabin.

## August 19

The plane landed late at Heathrow, I arrived at my hotel late and slept well into this morning. It's mid-afternoon now. I've shuttled from Heathrow to Gatwick and I'm ready to board a plane that will take me to Lilongwe, Malawi. Once in the air and flying south, I look out my porthole at the full moon hanging over the monster wing of the plane. I gaze at her and make a wish for a safe landing. The British pilot asks everyone to take their seats because we're heading into a "rough patch" and in his British accent he drawls that it will take nine hours to reach our destination. Do all pilots drawl?

## August 20

It must be around 4:30 in the morning. Most of the passengers are asleep. My porthole shade has been up all night so I could press my face into the cool plastic and watch the stars as we pushed through the black sky. I've no idea what direction we're flying now. Not long ago the moon passed over us heading westward home toward Barry and Rosie. If, as I suspect, we're flying south, I'll be able to watch the sunrise. Physical discomfort, excitement and lack of a soft pillow have made for fitful sleeping at best. Outside the sky is lightening—the long night is over at last.

The indigo bowl above me grows increasingly paler and a thin blue line stretches beneath a low bank of clouds. Two persistent stars linger high in the sky and are dimly reflected in the wing of the plane. How enormous is this space! As the gray sky blends into blue, the rising sun erases the stars. Salmon clouds bleach to pale yellow on the horizon below and dissipate upward into the blue-gray dome. A dirty blanket of cloud lounges ominously immediately below my wing obscuring the earth. I see no mountains, streams, deserts or lights and wonder if this featureless landscape is water we're flying over. The sky has turned as blue as my grandbaby's eyes.

It's now five o'clock in the morning and the dull steel of my wing has turned pink. Suddenly we change direction and the glittering sun pops over the forward edge of the wing as the plane dips like a monstrous bird tipping its head to better see the earth. When the plane rights itself, I close my eyes against the brilliant light and all sorts of colors and shapes dance and sparkle behind my lids. My porthole faces east now and it's the only one open to the morning. I'm thinking it's a miracle we're flying so high in this enormous sky and that this motley microcosm of humanity is still in the air hurtling into Africa.

## August 23

My intrepid friend did, indeed, meet me at the airport and we spent the next few of days mustering her out of the Peace Corps and catching up after two years apart.

Today we begin our safari and board a local flight to Zimbabwe, where we'll spend three days at an elephant camp. Since arriving in Lilongwe the worries stopped, but today just as we're about to board I learn that Malawi airlines forbids butane and possession of such is punishable by who knows what. I have two cordless curling irons stashed in my luggage, each powered by butane. American and British airlines have no such prohibition. I'd felt relieved by my "aha" discovery of cordless curling irons, which made scarce electricity on safari irrelevant. What happens now if I'm found out? This concern takes center stage, even edging out my fear of flying in a third-world, uninspected airplane. I decide to play dumb, stuff the curling iron in my camera bag and march through customs with as much bravado as I can muster. No one stops me. Then I wonder if there's a good reason for this rule on this particular airline and might my butane-filled curling irons blow up the plane. Joy is sick of my musings and tells me so. Fortunately our plane lands safely in Harare, where we're met by a driver who takes us into a city beset with political unrest and violence. We'll hole up here in a safe hotel for the night before moving to the camp.

## August 24

The elephant camp is located a half hour's drive from Victoria Falls and after driving for some time through government-owned land, we turn onto a dirt track leading to a private reserve, which is home to a herd of wild elephants as well as a small group of trained animals who've been rescued as babies from the guns of poachers. Immediately when we arrive at the lodge, we're offered a cold fruit drink and are ushered onto a terrace where a table is laid with a sumptuous lunch beneath the shade of a jacaranda tree and surrounded by a border of bright yellow flowers. A strip of lawn gives way to a flat vista of sand and scrub in the midst of which is a water hole where six elephants slosh water into their trunks and spray themselves. Awestruck, I'm unable to eat and rush to find my camera stashed with our luggage in the lodge. Just as I return, the elephants stroll off and in their place, a family of warthogs trots onto the lawn to nibble grass. Finally, I succumb to hunger and sit down with Joy and our hosts.

When we're finished eating, we're escorted to our round hut some distance from the lodge. Joy and I are eager to explore our living quarters. Two twin beds dressed in white are draped with mosquito netting and in an alcove behind a low interior wall, the bathroom is outfitted with a shower, fluffy towels and amenities befitting the Ritz. Above a circular, mahogany, knee-high wall, canvas and mosquito netting curtains are rolled up and we can see the nearby water hole and in the distance, a green and gold landscape. A lovely, cool, breeze blows through the large room and there's no need for the ceiling fan hanging from the thatched roof. With the netting and canvas rolled up we have an unobstructed view of the elephants who at this moment are tiptoeing past our hut to the watering hole. I'm beside myself with excitement. It's winter here in Zimbabwe, which explains the crisp, brown leaves on some of the trees, but there are others that remain evergreen and paint the landscape with soft green and bright yellow leaves. No mosquitoes this time of year.

Instead of being driven in a Land Rover to see the local wildlife, this afternoon we'll ride elephants under the careful supervision of their handlers. They carry folks on two games drives a day and when they're done, the elephants are free to browse in the bush and play in their mud wallow. If one strays too far afield, the handler whistles and the animal comes back. For the life of me, I don't know why. Such a large, intelligent animal could just as easily do as it pleased. Joy decides to take a nap and I head off to find the elephants. When I arrive at the paddock they're ready and saddled. I climb onto a tall platform and hoist myself astride Miss Ellie. I'd imagined having to spread my legs into an ungodly angle to accommodate the animal's broad back, but am pleasantly surprised to find the saddle is quilted and made in such a way that sitting is comfortable. Ahead of me, perched between Miss Ellie's huge, rough ears is her handler, Yanni, who commands her to join the parade of four loaded elephants making their way out of the enclosure and onto a red clay track bordered by soft, wheat-colored grasses, thornbushes and strewn with loose rocks.

Miss Ellie, known as a mischief, swipes trunkfuls of leaves whenever she can reach them and stuffs them in her mouth. Now and again she veers off the trail to find tastier fare in spite of Yanni's commands to the contrary. She walks on tiptoes as all elephants do and her footfalls make almost no sound as she steps slowly and purposefully over the rocky terrain. The only sounds I hear are the soft voices of the handlers talking to their elephants and the scraping of thorny branches against the animals' thick hide. After a while we stop at a swampy pool where the elephants slurp gallons of water into their trunks and squirt it into their mouths. I wait for a drenching, but it doesn't happen. I love my elephant.

## August 25

This morning I walk with the guide who's leading the game drive because I desperately need the exercise. Striding ahead of the convoy of four elephants, my host R. looks spiffy with blond hair poking out beneath the brim of his outback-style hat. A khaki shirt and shorts set off his tanned limbs. To complete the exotic picture, R. carries a lethal looking rifle causally slung across his back. Uncomfortable in the presence of any kind of weapon, I inquire about the rifle. R. tells me a month ago he was leading another game drive like ours and a lioness charged him. Taken by surprise and before he'd even had time to pull his rifle out of its sling, the lioness thought better of her intention and veered off into the bush with two cubs trailing behind her. I certainly hadn't thought of that possibility and here I'm on foot with a slow-draw guide. I stay close to R. for the remainder of the walk and try to forget about dangerous mother lions—and would have, if R. hadn't warmed to the subject of perilous encounters. Another reason for the rifle, he says, is to warn off wild elephants who like to cause trouble with their tamer cousins. Still, I feel remarkably safe around these half-wild, half-domesticated elephants, perhaps because they aren't predators by nature and are extraordinarily intelligent animals.

Just off the trail a pair of giraffes stands as tall as the thorn trees they've buried their heads in to bite off succulent leaves—not at all disturbed by the passage of the elephants and their baggage. Where the bush opens onto grassy places, impala graze and flick their short tails, staring at us as we go by. They're endlessly on the lookout for predators and one keeps watch while the others eat. Warthogs seem more distressed than the other animals at our approach and scuttle out of thickets looking silly with their pigtails sticking straight in the air. Exquisitely colored birds flit in and out of the scrub. The lilac-breasted roller, no larger than a robin is dressed in aqua and lilac. Everywhere we see red-billed hornbills that have large, thick, red, beaks and are handsomely garbed in black and white plumage. Little birds like bee-eaters sport iridescent feathers, which glint in the early morning sunlight. The carmine bee-eater is a brilliant red except for his blue-green head and light blue rump. Sunbirds burst in and out of the thornbushes like flashes of metallic green flames. So many birds—weavers decorate an entire tree with a community of hanging nests looking like Christmas ornaments, spoonbills, storks and glossy starlings tickle my imagination with their exotic names and eye-popping colors.

We return to the lodge just as the sun bears down and begins to cook us. We settle under the shade of the jacaranda and dig into an elaborate brunch. When we're done Joy and I return to our hut to read and nap. Unable to relax, I go out to the garden to chase warthogs with my camera until R. finds me and says the elephants will soon be going to the water hole for their mud baths. When the time comes, Yanni stops at our hut and we follow Miss Ellie and her friends as they make their way to the water. Watching elephants play in their bath is a joyous experience and their exuberance is as catching as laughter can be. First they spray themselves thoroughly, then each other before plopping down in the soupy water where they roll and flop with abandon like toddlers. When the bath and playtime are over, these huge beasts haul their shiny, mud-covered selves out of the wallow and amble into the bush to browse. We stay with the elephants until it's time for them to return to their shelter for the night and for us to get ready for dinner.

We're treated to a multicourse, candlelit dinner with the staff—we're the only guests tonight. When we're done one of the trainers invites us to accompany him while he doses a young orphan with antibiotics. The little elephant had been found a month ago with his foot clamped in a snare. The special care he's receiving has gone a long way to healing the ugly wound and in a short time, the baby has begun to learn some basic commands. He takes the mixture of medicine without complaint. We say goodnight and turn our lanterns to the path back to the lodge. Tomorrow morning we leave for Botswana.

## August 26

I didn't sleep well last night and have awakened with a stomachache. I feel just plain awful. Declining breakfast I took something to settle my stomach, but it's done little to help and I'm working hard to keep myself together during the endless van ride from Victoria Falls to Kasane, Botswana, where upon arrival we must board a very small plane, which seats four passengers and a "bush pilot." We take off into the wind and proceed on a wobbly, precarious flight to the King's Pool safari camp. Here we're met by a strange-looking, topless vehicle. Since this morning I've been deep breathing and focusing all my energy on controlling my mind and body's urges to evacuate. So far I've been successful.

Our long hot, dusty journey ends at the safari camp and immediately I take to bed in our luxurious canvas hut. Joy joins the afternoon game drive and I drift off to sleep. Suddenly, I'm awakened by thunderous trumpeting. Shaking the sides of the tent, elephants crash through the shrubs just outside its flimsy screen door and from the branches of the knob thorn trees above, baboons shriek insults at the retreating elephants. Baboons make an ungodly racket, sometimes for no reason at all, which may be either a curse or a blessing if they warn of intruders like hippos or lions. Napping is no longer possible. As I'm writing, a gleeful bunch of monkeys plays trampoline on the canvas above my head. Nearby the hippos tune up in the oxbow-shaped pool in the Linyanti River where they've lounged submerged, but for their nostrils, during the hottest hours of the day. Roused by the commotion, they fill the air with their peculiar barking laughter. We've been warned not to venture out at night without an escort because lions have been skulking around the compound and hippos come out of the pool to graze on the dry grasses around the tents. Hippos have a reputation for being irritable and unfriendly beasts; given how enormous they are, I'm skeptical about how our escorts can protect us armed with only a flashlight and a stick.

## August 27

I'm awake before daybreak. Most of the night sleep was elusive and fitful at best, interrupted, as it was by mysterious grunts, snorts and snuffles edging closer and closer around our tent. The baboons spent the night screaming invectives down at the hippos grazing under their trees and the hippos responded with barks sounding like bullhorns. As Joy and I walk to the lodge for an early breakfast I notice lion and elephant tracks in the sandy path. Last night's mysteries aren't so mysterious now.

We're off on a game drive and climb into a sideless, topless safari vehicle that makes its way down a sandy track into the mopane forest. A spotter sits in a seat attached to the front bumper and signals our driver to stop when a family of elephants led by a large female trailing a small baby steps quietly out of the bush and crosses the track in front of us giving us cautious sidelong glances. I snap several photographs of the elephant family until the matron trumpets to her family to move quickly and they melt into the thick brush. Then an adolescent straggler pushes through the shrubbery. Flapping large ears, he screams a warning at us. After making several halfhearted charges, he too crosses the track to follow in the wake of his family. I'm not used to elephants being so skittish and wonder why these are behaving in this manner.

Further down the trail we stop to watch four fat lionesses sprawled in the sun along the marshy banks of the Linyanti River. Their engorged bellies heave as they digest last night's meal. The cats barely acknowledge our presence. By now the sun is blisteringly hot and the game drive comes to an end. The animals have sought the shade of acacia or knobthorn trees where the dry breeze cools them and we return to the lodge to cool ourselves in the shade of the veranda where a huge buffet has been laid out for the guests. Just below the deck the river pool is filled with a pod of half-submerged hippos lolling about like a pile of shiny brown boulders. One of them lifts his head out of the water, opens his great toothy jaws and barks setting off a chorus of funny honking that never fails to make me giggle at the strangeness of hippo talk.

Deciding against the afternoon game drive, Joy and I spend a peaceful time in a hide a few hundred yards down a boardwalk from the lodge. We'd had to be escorted to this gazebo and were given a two-way radio should we need something. I wonder why we need the escort in broad daylight but keep my mouth shut. The hide is outfitted with two comfortable wicker chairs. Its thatched roof protects us from the hot afternoon sun and its open sides allow the breeze coming off the river to keep us comfortable. We're surrounded by tall papyrus and the river banks are lined with reeds, which sing and glitter in the slanting light when a breeze brushes through them. At the tip of a dead tree reaching its bony branches into the sky, two little bee-eaters, the size of warblers, sit so close to one another I can barely tell there are two. They're brilliantly dressed in iridescent green with yellow throats and orange bellies.

The sun has begun to set and tinges the papyrus gold. Above us the sky is still pale blue and cloudless. In a moment of restlessness inspired by an urge to find the nearby outhouse, I leave the hide. Just as I reach my destination I hear branches snapping and a large shape ambles out of the thick mopane scrub behind our hide. An enormous elephant heads toward the meadow by the river. Forgetting my mission I race back to the hide to get my camera and there are three more bull elephants wading into the river to drink and spray themselves. When they're done they slowly cross the meadow and stop near a copse of thornbushes where two of the boys begin to wrestle one another. The air reverberates with the clanking of tusks and loud trumpeting just as the massive orange sun drops below the horizon. We call for our escort.

Awaiting the dinner hour, I hear a familiar spine-tingling groan outside our tent. Then all's quiet—not even a baboon breaks the silence. Later at dinner, we're told two male lions had passed close by our tent. Needless to say, I'm inordinately grateful for our escorts and to think, tomorrow morning I've signed up for a walking game drive with a small-armed guide.

## *August 28*

All packed for the afternoon journey to our final destination, Joy and I get up at dawn to make ready for this morning's walk. After a fruity breakfast, she and I and three other women head into the bush accompanied by not one but three guides, two of whom are armed with rifles. Just outside the compound our group follows an elephant's footprints in the sandy track—each impression is as large as a pie plate. My sandaled feet leave deeper prints in the sand than do these elephantine feet. Somewhere I read that because elephants walk on their tiptoes, their tread is silent and soft enough to leave only the slightest impression. I've noticed when I hear an elephant approach it's usually because I can hear the barely audible rumble she uses to talk to her family or I hear the splintering of twigs as the animal bushwhacks through the forest or the cracking of branches being ripped off trees—never her footfalls.

The elephant we're following keeps to the track and is leaving a trail of sticky fluid in the sand. It's likely it's a male in musth who's ready to mate and who may be feisty and irritable. In a while his footprints disappear into the mopane forest where herds of elephants have leveled trees or broken them until the landscape looks like acres and acres of shoulder-high shrubs, broken tree trunks and dead windfalls. We follow the still-visible tracks and come upon a small clearing where the bleached bones of an elephant lie scattered about amidst huge piles of dung and numerous large footprints. Had our male come to pay his respects as others had done?

We pay ours and continue to follow him along a game trail to a drying water hole where several impala, a scruffy herd of zebra and a family of baboons mill about until they catch our scent on the wind and disappear into the thickets. Skirting the water hole, our guide motions for us to be quiet and stay close. Our bull elephant—the one in whose footprints I'd been stepping—stands sixty meters upwind from where we're partially hidden in the scrub, contentedly pulling up trunkfuls of dry golden grass and stuffing it into his mouth. We watch for a while, taking photographs until it's time to head back to the lodge for lunch. We leave the elephant in peace.

As we make slow progress down the deep sandy track I spot a tiny carmine bee-eater perched on the branch of a thorn tree. He's so red it's startling. The bird follows our little parade for a moment and flies away flaring his long tail behind him.

After lunch Joy and I load our gear into a safari vehicle and take our seats behind the driver who'll deliver us to our next destination. We pass the bull elephant standing alone by the water hole we'd just come from this morning. Further down the road there are more elephants far across an expanse of low growing scrub. One of them raises its head, flaps its ears and begins to walk toward our vehicle, which is struggling to push forward in the sand. In front of us a large tree lies across the road. We stop, unable to move forward. Ragged stumps on either side of the track block our passage around the fallen tree. With my camera at the ready I turn to see the elephant walking very fast and gaining on us. Shaking her head, she flaps her ears as if in a mock charge. She rents the air with a roar and it becomes quite evident this elephant isn't pretending, she's on a mission to do us harm. While walking is the only gait an elephant has, an angry or frightened animal can reach a powerful stride of twenty-five miles per hour. This one is gaining on us rapidly and we're stuck. Trailing behind the charging matron is a small baby who's barely able to keep up with its mother.

Just as our driver shifts into reverse hoping to find a way through the maze of stumps, the elephant drives her tusks through the rear steel panel of the truck and into the backseat. When she backs up for another charge, the driver stomps on the accelerator and we bounce precariously over the stumps and crash through the underbrush until we skid back onto the track. Undeterred by our getaway, the elephant pursues us. Several yards ahead another tree blocks the road. This time we're able to get around it easily and speed away, leaving the matron behind trumpeting her anger.

Once safely at our destination two of us—the driver and I—climb down out of the truck to look at the damage. Joy thinks the whole matter is a delicious adventure and denies the slightest tremble at the thought of what might have happened. Two large holes have been gouged at an angle through the steel plate behind the rear seat. It looks like this elephant intended to overturn us, and it also seems she deliberately knocked down the trees to bar our way. Later that afternoon we hear the track has been closed to safari traffic and I'm told that just across the border between Botswana and Namibia poachers, driving vehicles much like ours, frequently kill elephants for their ivory tusks. This explains the mother elephant's rage when she spotted us from across the mopane scrubland.

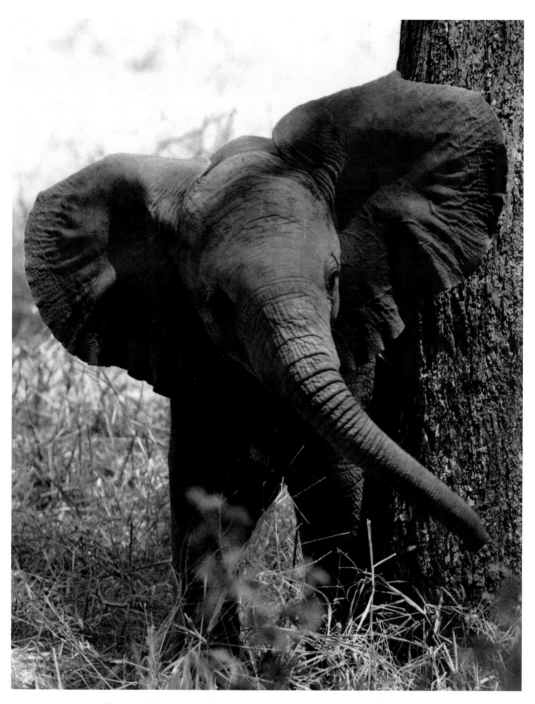

"Our first teacher is our own heart."

⌒ *Cheyenne saying*

It's late afternoon when we arrive at Savuti camp and after a cold fruit drink we're escorted to our tent. The Savuti Game Reserve is noted for its large population of lions and a pride of lionesses has been camping out here for several days. Hot and tired and ready for a long shower, Joy and I decide against the afternoon game drive. We've had enough adventure for the day, and besides the sun is still high and scalding. We stay cool in the shelter of our tent where a dry breeze wafts through the mosquito netting. Our open-to-the-air accommodations consist of a tent covered with a thatched roof, its canvas sides fastened to a wooden platform perched on the edge of a low embankment overlooking a large pan—a meadow-like basin, which collects summer rains and holds an ever-shrinking body of water well into the dry winter season. Bounded by forest and scrubland the small pool attracts lions, elephants and game animals that meander out of the forest and low gray thickets to drink at the only water hole for miles around, which lies a couple of hundred yards from our tent. I take a deep breath and fill my lungs with the fragrance of drying herb grasses. I'm ready for a shower.

The bathroom, built like a stall, is situated outside the screen door down a mahogany gangway. Two and a half of its walls are made of horizontal mahogany strips and the front opens onto an unobstructed view of the golden landscape and the water hole. In spite of its rustic appearance, the small cubicle is outfitted with an exquisite tile sink, plush terry towels and robes hanging from brass hooks, soaps, shampoo and other amenities. Next to the pottery soap dish a miniature frog sits and watches intently as I make ready to bathe. I can't wait to wash the gritty layers of dust off my body. From the curtainless shower enclosure I can see two male lions strolling over to the water hole closely followed by the safari truck, which rolls into camera range of the animals. What a sight!

Then I remember I'm in the buff and within range of human eyes aided by binoculars. Now it's entirely too disturbing to remain where I am, so I don a terry robe and wait for them to leave. When the coast is clear, I luxuriate in the warm spray. Wrapped again in velvety white terry cloth, I sit on our tiny veranda to dry just as a bull elephant makes his dignified way across the meadow to drink. In a moment, two lionesses shamble out of a thicket to the right of our camp. I'm filled with amazement at my circumstances here. It's hard to believe I'm seeing all this wildlife so close by and in the comfort of such elegant quarters.

After a lavish multicourse dinner accompanied by wine and dessert, Joy and I are escorted back to our tent to prepare for tomorrow's departure and a very long journey via South Africa to London before flying home. I repair to the bathroom to wash my face and brush my teeth. Just as I squeeze toothpaste onto the brush, there's a deafening groan nearby, followed by growls. All sorts of images flash through my mind and feeling completely unprotected, I gather up my kit and run into the tent as quickly as I can. The moonless night feels particularly dark. In spite of a sky filled with millions of stars, I can't see a thing beyond the walkway. Slamming the flimsy screen door behind me I leap into bed just as a lion grunts bringing on a prideful of roaring that sends a shudder through my bones. In my haste I've forgotten to turn off the generator-powered bathroom light. There's no way I'll go back.

The tent feels fragile and vulnerable to the possible attack of starving lions that are just waiting to claw through the filmy mosquito netting in hopes of finding a delectable meal. Now there's silence. In minute or two the bellowing begins again. Joy listens and says, "Isn't it thrilling?" and rolls over to fall sound asleep.

I lie rigid in my bed, wide awake and breathing fast. The roaring stops and silence fills the space with suspense. With nothing better to do, I time the racket, which swells to a crescendo matching my heartbeat and peters out with a few grunts. The earsplitting, bone-rattling bellows begin at twenty-minute intervals. I recall reading that when lions mate, the male carries on his conjugal attacks every twenty minutes or so for hours until he's satisfied his genetic material has been safely deposited. Convinced there's an orgy going on outside our tent, I suspect the male lion I saw this afternoon has come out of the shadowy bush to visit the girls hanging around our camp. He's chosen one as his bride and the others cheer the pair on. These thoughts bring some relief, but not for long.

I'd hoped that last night's fitful sleep interrupted by screaming baboons, laughing hippos and Lariam dreams might have tired me out enough to sleep through most anything, but it's not to be. My imagination crouches in the darkest African night summoning up a kaleidoscope of disturbing images. I'm convinced when their sexual appetites are satisfied, the lions will be famished and will prowl through the camp eager in search of dinner. How easy it would be to find it close at hand and trapped in a tent. And now I have to pee! I'll be damned if I'm going out to the toilet alone. I could arm myself with the air horn with which each tent is equipped and which is to be used strictly for medical emergencies and fire. Roaring lions on the threshold of one's sleeping quarters isn't on the list. Still, I've decided if a lion merely taps at the door, I'll let loose with the horn no matter the consequences. My problem is solved when Joy wakes and needs to use the bathroom too. I follow close on her heels threatening bodily harm if she leaves me alone with the lions. Once safely back in bed I force my breathing to slow and meditate on my grandbaby and Rosie until finally, I drift off into a light sleep. A short while later, around two o'clock, the exhausted lions stop their terrible noise.

## August 29

Today we leave on our journey home. We're packed and ready to go, but not before one last game drive. Except for a few impalas, the landscape is quiet and empty of animal life until we come upon a pride of fat-bellied sleeping lionesses stretched out on the grassy savannah in the warming sun. I lean out of the safari vehicle to get a closer photograph of these lovely, tawny cats who now look so benign, I want to touch one.

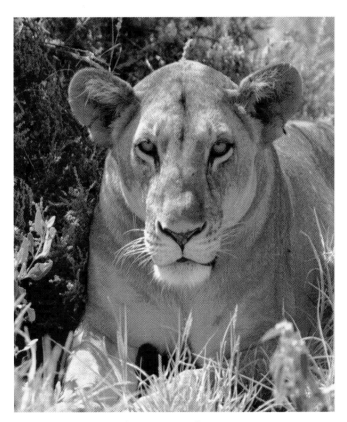

## *The Feral Cat*

Under a mottled sky
there's a feral cat
coiled in tall grass,
drowsing—gold eyes slit to watch.
Abandoned to wildness she waits;
sniffs green air for finches red as raspberries
until hunger draws knives from her paws.
She springs. A blue jay breaks the air
with a cry. A sparrow's feather
is all there is
sometimes
it's not time to die.
Hunger still rakes her belly.

And me—I cheer for the bird.
Yet no less ravenous than the cat
I'm loath to concede a hunger wild as this.

# Prey and Predator

In this world, in one way or another, everybody is armed and dangerous. Nature's armamentarium is filled with razor teeth, fangs, talons, knife-like beaks, arrows, sucking mouths, poisons, germs, guns and missiles. All the rawness of nature is played out on a grand scale on Africa's plains, savannas, deserts and woodlands. Baboons smile and flash their sharp incisors, hyena jaws are so strong their teeth can crush bone, lions use their claws like sabers to bring down their prey and inside the bulbous jaws of hippopotami are huge tusks for piercing enemies and teeth for masticating grasses. Some snakes sport fangs oozing with venom and others have mouths so huge they swallow prey larger than themselves. And some predators are so small they're invisible to the naked eye. In Africa the seeming lawlessness of living and dying isn't diluted by the pretensions of human civilization; here living and dying is unvarnished.

On safari one experiences a wild world long lost to other than the most inhospitable parts of the earth. The continent's vast beauty, its diverse landscapes and wild creatures are nowhere else to be found in such magnificence and in such multitudes. Following a long colonial tradition of trophy hunting, now prohibited, tourists today come to witness a kill. Guides scan the plains for feeding animals and when sighted, a covey of vehicles will race to surround a pride of lions feasting on the bloody carcass of a hapless zebra and all you hear is the chomping of jaws and the whirr of video cameras and clicking shutters. A visitor will be especially thrilled when the rare opportunity arises to watch a cheetah chase an impala to the ground.

I'm not sure what it is that draws us to the kill. Are we imbued with a deeply carnivorous instinct, an ancient drive we humans prefer to deny? I know every living body on this earth, every creature who crawls, walks, swims or flies or just is, is a predator and I know we'll all be prey to one predator or another at one time or another. Much as I'm discomfited by the knowledge, I'm the ultimate predator sitting as I do at the top of the food chain. But even I'll be someone's

132

prey, perhaps to another cancer cell, a virus, a bacterium, a mosquito, a tick, another human or a hungry lioness.

Killing on the plains of Africa isn't frivolous, isn't evil—it's about life. Animals kill, if they must, to fight rivals for suitable mates to ensure the continuity of their gene pool. They vie for territory in which to gather food, often in scarce supply, and to find homes where they can raise their young in safety. One minute a pride of lionesses tears at the flank of an antelope, the next the girls bathe in the sun dappled grass and play like house cats with their rambunctious cubs. Nurturing the hope of their species, most females don't indulge in gratuitous violence in spite of the brutality of the slaughter. Nature may appear pragmatic and cruel when one thinks that only the fittest survive, but rooted as it is, deep in the grand design, the taking of life to give life to another is neither vengeful nor capricious.

It's the human predator I fear most because we take predation far beyond nature's drive to perpetuate life. We murder creatures not only for food, but often for the sake of killing, for vengeance, for a trophy or for some perceived benefit to ourselves. Even when our basic needs for food, shelter and the opportunity to procreate have been satisfied, we prey on those who're different from us in race and ideology and worse, we destroy each other in the name of God. In our efforts to create a world in our image we appear to be on the brink of distorting nature's fundamental processes by altering the environment, destroying habitats, displacing people and animals, hastening their extinctions as if they were worthless. It's true, I'm far removed from nature's rawness and I often deny my deepest, forgivable instincts. I don't see myself as a predator, a thief of land or a destroyer of the environment I love and yet, in many ways, I am. I don't kill fish to eat salmon, I live on land already stolen from someone else and I'm less green than I should be.

In spite of our baser drives, we humans are also driven by a desire for transcendence and community. I struggle to find that place where I can own my natural self, the part of me that cares first for my own life and gratifying my basic needs and the self that yearns to live gracefully with the messiness of life and still find meaning in that struggle in a complicated and often dangerous world. Walking around the bog and its meadows or through the quiet forest, nature's violence is nearly invisible—she mops up after herself with great speed. The rotting sunfish on the bank of the pond disappears after a day; I don't see the fox return to her den with a rabbit clamped in her jaws.

I'm exquisitely aware that the cycle, of which I'm a part, carries on with or without me and that I'm part of a grand plan designed millions of years ago, no less than the animals who do what they must to live. I avoid violence as much as possible while trying to accept its inevitability. I don't travel to Africa to witness a kill but to see her babies. Yet understanding nature's version of prey and predator in the raw helps me to make sense of my own human nature, of my original animal nature and how it's changed, been improved upon or degraded. Witnessing the hard scrabbling for survival in the wild places of Africa forces me to accept nature's version and to be more cognizant of my impact on the creatures and on the land in which I live. While I grapple with my fears and learn to trust life more fully and realistically, I come a little closer to accepting my place in the inescapable cycle of living and dying and the knowledge that one day I will be prey to something.

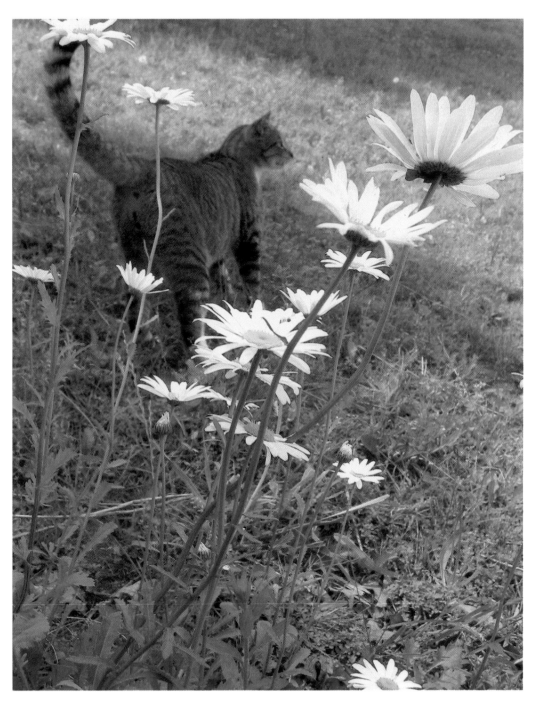

"There are no ordinary cats."

*Colette*

135

# September

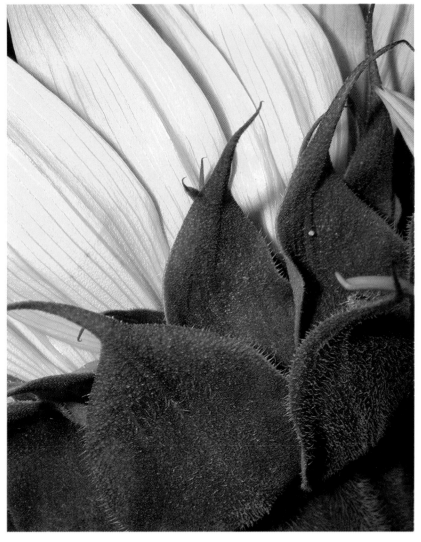

"Earth laughs in flowers."
*Ralph Waldo Emerson*

# September Journal

*September 9*

I'm happy to be home and walking the bog again with Rosie. The cranberry meadow looks like a green velvet carpet, but sadly the small meadows are still stressed. Herbicides have browned the wildflowers and sometimes when the wind is right, a pungent chemical odor blots out late summer's herbal aromas. As we make our way around the perimeter of the bog there are few signs of wildlife—no butterflies because there aren't any wildflowers. The geese have disappeared again and the songbirds are silent. A few dragonflies zip by us and two shiny crows caw from an old birch leaning over the shadowy edge of the upper pond where a heron fishes. Nevertheless, the weather has been lovely and cool since I arrived home and the nights are downright chilly. Swamp maples are just beginning to turn color and their rosy hues soften the barren landscape.

At home the feeders hang full of seed. I wonder if the fall migration has begun early or have the birds found their wild harvest preferable to the canned stuff I offer? After one last visit, yesterday, the hummingbirds left for the south, and I suspect the redwings and many of the summer sparrows have departed with them. The dreary silence is relieved by the liquid notes of a lone Carolina wren who sings from her hiding place in the thick foliage of the wisteria vine outside my window. She's accompanied by goldfinches clinging to the thistle feeders murmuring softly to one another. I sorely miss the company of my other winged friends and the flurry greeting me when I enter the house.

I've been learning about migration and found out that little birds like wrens and warblers prefer to migrate in the safety of darkness, while large birds such as geese and hawks will travel with impunity during daylight hours. Monarchs and common green darner dragonflies will join the birds on their southward journey later this month. I'm in awe of warblers and hummingbirds who fly incredible distances, sometimes across an ocean without rest. But even more amazing are the fragile butterflies and dragonflies who migrate into the winds and weathers that beset them along their journey. Such courage! I shall be thinking of these small travelers when I'm next in the air filled with anxiety.

Late in the afternoon Rosie and I go across the street into the cornfield where the cornstalks have been chopped up for silage leaving rows and rows of stubble. A large flock of starlings soars in formation across the field and like a falling kite, they swoop into the bony branches of a dead maple dressing the tree with dark iridescent, noisy leaves. Along the roadside green milkweed pods fatten and I'm waiting for their silky seeds to burst from their confines and fill the air with rainbow-lit filaments.

## September 18

Still no songbirds; even the residents are quiet. Cicadas buzz during the day and crickets chirp in the evening. Down at the bog Rosie and I startle a small flock of geese afloat on the pond. They drift away from us chattering noisily. They've come back to glean corn kernels from the shorn fields. Rounding the eastern edge of the cranberry meadow, I smell the special tart fragrance of ripe grapes that fills the air where bunches of midnight-purple clusters of fruit hang from vines woven too high into the bordering trees to reach. Years ago I filled grocery bags with wild grapes, boiled them, then strained the mixture and thickened it with sugar until it turned to jelly. I haven't tasted such deliciously tangy, wild and sweet jelly since.

The sky is deep iris-blue and dotted with bunches of clouds. A sparrow flits out of a shrub growing near the trail. I'm astonished by the tenacity of a life force that's urged a clump of purple asters to push their way up through a mat of mowed grasses after being razed earlier this summer, determined to bloom in their season to make seed for next year. The farmer hasn't a chance of winning his battle with "weeds" after all—no matter how many herbicides or insecticides or how often the meadows are shorn, there'll always be a stubborn, errant daisy, a hardy bug and persistent grasses who'll return in the spring to reproduce. It's happening now at summer's end and I'm less discouraged knowing this about nature.

## September 19

Now that we're entering another cycle, a season of dormancy, I'm reflecting on dying—living and dying and the future. Last night I forced myself to watch a Bill Moyers' documentary about dying "On Our Own Terms." People talked frankly about their terminal illnesses and their feelings about dying. Much to Barry's dismay, I've spent the last four evenings watching this program convinced I need to learn, to know how I'd like the process to go for me when I'm faced with death myself. For me the stark reality of dying sends a stomach-twisting dose of fear through me and I know it's naive, perhaps even arrogant, of me to think I might prepare myself for a "good death" but somehow the thinking gives me a strange sense of control.

I know the reality challenges one's courage and faith, but I also wonder if one is supposed to keep fear quietly under one's wing if one is to die a good death. The truth is I don't picture myself going "gently into that good night" without a big fuss. Concern for my performance? What a concept. What I'm really afraid of is suffocation, inexorable and unrelieved pain and abandonment. I know what an extraordinary act of love and patience it is to be with a loved one who's dying. I refuse to drown in these disturbing musings, but I don't want to shrink from considering them either, because thoughts of my mortality remind me each day is a precious gift. Staying in the moment is a tricky juggling act—not focusing too long on the future and still preparing for it as best as I can. So here I am, ripening with the asters, the milkweed and the changing leaves in this season of maturation and looking toward winter without trepidation at least for now.

Small family groups of Canada geese fly low over the reddening cranberry meadow until a flotilla of birds congregates on the pond to preen and gossip. Where the trail sides were bare only a few weeks ago, goldenrod has pushed its way up through the fading spires of purple loosestrife along the banks of the upper pond—its arrow-shaped clusters of miniature, yellow blossoms glow in the afternoon sun. A few ragged water lilies still bloom, but most have closed up and sunk to the bottom of the pond. It's a miracle how more and more wildflowers have popped up again to bloom along the bog trail—ragweed and daisy-flowered mayweed mixes with yellow goatsbeard and yellow hawkweed. Lavender clusters of common fleabane, each flower a tiny golden disk ringed with petals bloom nearby their cousins the asters. The aster, Greek for star, is aptly named and nestled among the fading stalks of joe-pie weed, they look like a sky full of stars. Rosie's tail is matted with burrs growing at the wood's edge.

On the way home from the bog a soft wing noise high up in an oak catches my attention. A young red-tailed hawk lands on a branch, settles his wings and tips his head to the road to watch us pass beneath him before flying further down the road. I think he finds easy prey in the abundance of chipmunks darting incautiously in and out of the stone walls, their mouths stuffed with acorns. Too often these days I find a hapless chipmunk flattened by a tire and I'm horrified when I'm forced to a screeching halt to let a panicked chipmunk decide whether or not to cross in front of me. The acorns are plentiful this season and Rosie and I dodge these little bullets dropping from the oaks and littering the roadside. I'd rather not have a shower of nuts rain on my car, or worse on my head. Some of the acorns drop on their own accord and some are nipped off their twigs by gray squirrels who race down the tree trunks to hide their harvest, sometimes in places they forget. In the spring these hidden nuts will crack and sprout under a protective layer of leaf litter. So happy to be walking, Rosie pretends to be deaf when I caution her not to eat acorns.

Later this afternoon, reclining in Barry's new chair reading, I look up from my book to find Rosie staring at me from her bed on the sofa. She holds my gaze and

I hers until she blinks first, then she stares again. What in the world is she thinking? Her brown eyes are peaceful, yet I sense she's trying to tell me something in this quiet moment we share. I glance at the clock and sure enough it's getting close to five and time for her supper. Many events have altered my life, not the least of which is sharing it with Rosie—Rosie and Patches.

Patches came to me first and in her cat-way soothed me when I needed it most and loved me when I needed loving. Then came Rosie, who from the beginning made it clear she wouldn't be a floor dog. She'd sleep as close to me as she could and if necessary share the space with Patches. Never tiring of our routine walks, Rosie teaches me every day how to be present to all that's around me. She sniffs the air with a wiggle of her nose, she hears rustling leaves and bounds after chipmunks. When she's in the mood for serious play, she grabs the largest stick she can hold in her mouth and prances around and around, lifting all four paws off the ground, levitating as if wearing air shoes. I want to dance the way she does with my feet barely touching the ground. Instead, she makes me laugh and I hug her and am rewarded with a wet kiss on the nose.

I talk to Rosie about a lot of things; sometimes its just chatter and sometimes I mull over problems. She listens with her soft ears cocked forward and I ground myself in her presence. I hear my voice with all its musicality, all its dissonance and harshness. I'm not embarrassed to reveal my deepest corners to Rosie—and when I do, my voice becomes clearer, less hesitant and my forays into the deeps become less frightening. Like a shadow, Rosie follows me from room to room until I come to rest and she lies at my feet. Still gazing at me, I tell her how much I love her and she dips her eyelids. For this single moment nothing else matters to me. I get up to make her supper.

Speaking of dark corners, once I kept a spotless house—at least on the surface; what couldn't be seen beneath the rug, behind the sofa, or under the refrigerator didn't matter, but a towel hung askew, a crummy countertop or footprints marring the velvety surface of a carpet caused me fits. These small messes no longer bother me and I wonder now if my compulsion for an orderly exterior masked the grimy, dusty interior of my soul? Peering into that dark place, noting its murderous, vicious thoughts or the piteous, dismal, suffering me has been a dangerous pastime. These cobwebbed corners are filled with distorted thinking, anger, alienation and abandonment and fear. There lurks the demon that accuses me of fakery and reminds me I have nothing worthwhile to say. There resides the demon who tells me when all is said and done, I'm exquisitely alone and someday won't exist at all. I try to imagine what it would be like not to be a body, a personality, a thought. I'm most afraid of losing one sense after another, little by little until my world shrinks to the size of an invalid's bed made small by illness. Having spent a lifetime's worth of energy blocking my ears against the demon's seductive rationalizations and fraudulent opinions, I've begun to dare to look into this dark self and while I've not befriended the treacherous side of myself, I've become less timid about treading into its unlit corners. There's more to me than the grim side.

These days my house isn't so tidy, but it's cleaner now that its darkest nooks and crannies are better lit. Scraping cat and dog fur off the bed each morning with a lint brush is only a minor chore when I've spent the night cavorting with animal souls in my dreams and Patches and Rosie warm my chilly nights. Moments of joy are less likely to sneak by me and I know I have the capacity to feel the peace my soul has craved. It's been all too easy to suffocate in my own gravity and as I grow older I'm honing my sense of the absurd, nonsensical bits of life so laughter comes more easily even in the midst of gloom.

### September 24

My writing lesson for the day is to write about a door key and I can't for the life of me think of anything, but here goes with letting thoughts just ramble and tumble out onto the paper. The first image suggested by a door key is of a large, heavy, brass key, which fit the antique lock to the door of the house in which I grew up. The key I use to let myself into my house today is also brass, but it's flimsy and lightweight. Most of our inside doors have keyless locks—not very interesting. Now I see doors, all locked, requiring just the right key to open them. Among them is a splendid, mysterious door invisible to my eyes, which needs a special key to unlock it, one that's not yet been designed. Sometimes I see the key and sometimes I lose it. New ideas, feelings all key-open doors in my mind—an intuition, a gesture by another being can unlock a door, just as this silly exercise has unlocked a small cabinet in my imagination. I've opened the door to my house with a brass key and then unlocked my mind.

It's been a quiet, cloud-filled day and the air heavy with moisture, sometimes spitting drizzle. Late this afternoon a patch of sunlight pokes out from behind a flying cloud. Rosie and I delayed our walk until the weather decided what it was going to do. A cool breeze has wiped away the last of the clouds and overturns the blushing leaves.

### September 27

When I awoke this morning, the air had a chilly edge to it. When I opened my eyes and stretched away the night's stiffness, I lay back and watched more clouds, this time white and billowy ones soar through the chicory sky overhead. Patches pats my cheek with her velvet paw and Rosie snores beside me.

A warm shaft of sunlight slants through the porch window and I sit listening to a solitary cricket chirrup inside the room. A great honking of geese drowns the cricket's song. Several families are heading for the cornfield. The air is perfectly still this afternoon and the sun slowly disappears into a gray-blue cloud. All of a sudden the wind freshens sending clouds tearing across the sky and a burst of rain ripples down the windows.

More and more maples have turned color. The edges of their leaves are on fire with a flame that will spread until whole trees turn scarlet and orange. Canada goose families are gathering down at the bog where the winterberry bushes are crimson with shiny fruit. The blue jays, who've been uncharacteristically quiet this summer, are squawking again in the woods. I love fall. It seems such a short season compared to the others. The brilliance of autumn quickly drifts northward until all but the evergreens have let loose their raiment to stand proud and naked to face winter. No longer do I mind the coming of winter. It's become a cleansing time, a part of life's roundness where my world is pared down to simple shapes and dark, muted colors. What appears to my eyes as drab senescence—branches gray like bones—is only preparation for another luscious journey, a birth, a blossoming, then a letting go and resting. I'm off to plant a bag of tulips I bought yesterday. I want to see what comes up next spring.

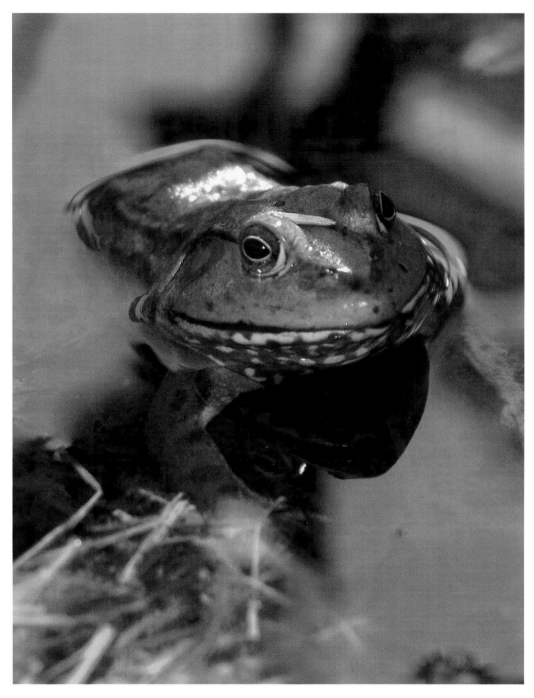

"Never a day passes but that I do myself
the honor to commune with some of
nature's varied forms."

*George Washington Carver*

## Sleep

The earth pirouettes around the sun
and morning light slides across my bed.
A blue wind dances through my window on curtained feet.
I rise out of the velvet fungus of sleep
where blurred images unreel in slow kaleidoscopic tricks;
where I'm the heroine whose unleashed dreams gamble with fantasy.

Still on the edge of sleep extravagant thoughts tumble
like swallows plunging across a plum sky:
On borrowed feet I run under a moon over dunes,
through shadows of moist grasses to the ocean's lip.
Here at the brink,
I lie like a cat with sleep trapped in her paws.

# Seasons of the Elm

It wasn't until I was five years old that I truly saw the solitary elm tree rising above the roof of the old colonial house in which I grew up. As much as I tried to hug its thick rough trunk, it was too big for my small arms to hold on to. From the dormer window in my bedroom I could watch this majestic tree change with the seasons. I was convinced the elm had sprouted out of its circle of lawn like a great fountain so that its gracefully drooping branches could cast dappled shadows on the grass. My mother told me the elm hadn't always been in the center of our driveway; it had first taken root and grown to adulthood in a nearby field on a farm she'd purchased just before I was born.

Even our house had been erected on another site than on the one it now sat. Having little patience with delaying gratification of her whims, my mother had the house lifted from its original stone foundation and the elm hoisted out of the earth and moved both to where she wanted them. This was no mean feat in those days. The spot she'd chosen to plant her house and her tree was in the center of a large parcel of pastureland in the middle of a rural neighborhood. Our property spread over fields, meadows, swamps and a forest and it was intersected by ancient, crumbling stone walls marking boundaries.

A long, yellow gravel driveway curved up from the narrow tar road and circled around the elm. I liked the way the small stones crunched underfoot and the way they sang under the tires of a car when it turned off the road and stopped under the old tree at our front door. I always knew when Nana was coming to visit long before I'd hear the brass doorknocker thwacking three times. The sounds of her tires crunching pebbles as she inched her ancient Nash up the driveway was unmistakable. Nana lived in a dark, mysterious, old-smelling Victorian house in the city and often came out to the country to visit us.

For some time the elm was the center of my small universe, a silent witness to the life unfolding in the house it sheltered and to the child whose dreams grew inside her year by year. The sturdy tree withstood droughts, it bowed and tossed in the howling winds, its branches bent with the weight of ice and snow and it even resisted the plague of Japanese beetles, which devastated the neighborhood elm population. My elm stood straight and tall.

When spring warmed the air and melted the snow in March the farm sprang to life; ewes dropped their lambs, the cows were released from their pens and with udders swinging and tails in the air, they kicked up their heels in the fresh pastures. My pony raced out the barn door into the paddock snorting and prancing with pleasure. We all came out of hibernation in March.

When spring peepers first began their loud chorus, I'd fly out of the winter confines of my house each morning to watch new grasses spike up from the brown thatch under the elm where daffodils were already poking their thick shoots up through the lawn. The elm let its tightly held buds pop open until each drooping branch was dressed in delicate, pale green lace. Early in April lying under the elm I was sure I could see each bud swelling until flowers burst open and leaves unfurled. I was intoxicated by the smell of warm dampness, of greening things and the pungent odor coming off the pastures where a winter's pile of cow dung had recently been spread. A pale carpet of timothy grass and alfalfa covered the fields. In late spring the elm's serrated leaves had turned deep green and the tree had become thick with life. Squirrels dashed up and down the massive trunk nattering and scolding, a robin made her nest and raised her brood in the crook of a high branch, tree frogs sang all night from its twigs and blue birds built their nest in the birdhouse my mother had nailed to elm's trunk.

My best friend lived across the field from my house and when she came to play with me, we'd lie on our bellies under the elm and each measure a square foot of turf to see who could identify the most flora and fauna there. We learned the names of bugs, wildflowers and innumerable birds. Whoever found the first four-leaf clover won something—I don't remember what. One year before the lawn was mowed, I came across a nest of baby rabbits hidden in the grass.

Letting the screen slam behind me on hot summer afternoons I went to the elm to lie in its cool shade and look up at the sky through its dense leaf canopy. Stretching my arm in the grass I'd let an ant crawl on my skin until I couldn't stand the tickle any longer. Summer days seemed endless then and yet they melted away and before I knew it the leaves of the elm had begun to yellow and the air had a familiar bite when I rose in the morning. I hated the sound of crumpling elm leaves under my sneakers and I didn't like the acrid smell of their burning because it meant summer's lazy days of exploration and dreaming were over. The first days of kindergarten, of first grade, fourth grade, tenth grade—all those first days of school in September, I hated.

When the snow began to fly, I was out under the elm to build a snowman. Rolling a snowball around and around until it was big enough for a belly, I set it against the trunk of the elm and rolled another into a head. When I was done, he'd have a carrot for a nose, pebbles for eyes, a twig for a mouth and an old straw hat on his head. Then I'd tumble in the snow to make flying angels waving my arms up and down. These snow angels were magical and did something mysterious when I went into the house and out of their sight. By the next morning, they'd disappeared. My mother filled a bird feeder hung from a low branch on the elm every day and every day it was emptied by dozens of blue jays, chickadees, sparrows, nuthatches and juncos.

Once I hung a small wooden feeder at my bedroom window and spent hours sticking my hand filled with sunflower seeds out of the open window to wait for a chickadee to land on a frozen finger and take a seed. I was overjoyed when a little bird finally did alight, grabbed a seed from my hand and flew off with it.

Over the years, through all the seasons, the old elm watched me grow from a small child to a lanky adolescent and bloom into a young woman. It heard my tears of frustration and hilarious laughter and finally it saw me drive down the golden driveway in a drenching October rainstorm with my new husband—a young woman filled with dreams and hopes and a blessing in her womb. This was to be the last time I looked back to see my weeping elm. A year later my mother sold our home. I wept for my life there on the farm and for my elm.

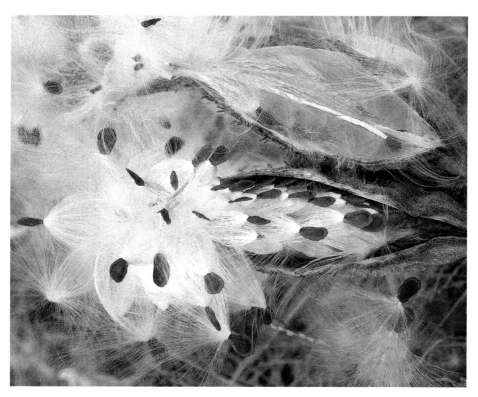

## No Time for Milkweed

I step on plants springing from broken places.
I don't see weeds;
not even a cluster of blushing flowers thrust at me,
exhaling perfume so sweet, even monarchs, red beetles and bees
halt their feverish flights.
There isn't time to let sticky milk bleed onto my finger from a velvet leaf.
Before the honeybee fills her saddlebags with pollen,
before the butterfly probes for nectar in a huddle of blossoms,
I'm away.
I can't wait for green and swelling pods to brown and burst and spill;
I'm off before the wind lofts seeds into the air
to float on silky filaments like a storm of elfin parachutes.
I'm gone before a tiny brown disk falls to clasp the earth
and coil its leg into the soil.
Before a delicate green spire lifts sunward, I'm long gone,
skidding across the seasons
as if one day
I'll stop.

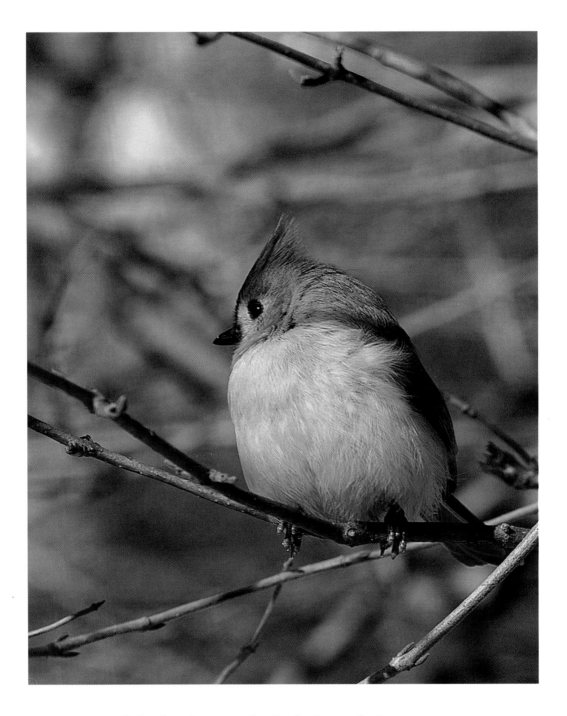

"The birds pour forth their souls in notes
of rapture from a thousand throats."
*William Wordsworth*

# In the Dark

*Thoughts on Waking in the Middle of the Night*

Here I am, eyes wide open and unable to go back to sleep. A square of moonlight shines down on me through the sky window like a comforter and I snuggle under it. I often think night was meant to be dark and mysterious and undiscovered by sleepers, but lying awake in this black velvet place I uncover recesses in my mind barely accessible in daylight. Asleep I'm happily oblivious to all those that slink, crawl, slither, prowl and stalk in the darkness. I'm unaware of sneaky nocturnal creatures shopping for prey, including my own thoughts. Waking in the middle of the night can throw me at the mercy of loneliness like no other time, especially when it feels as if I'm the only one awake—when even the mouse who scratches madly inside the wall at the foot of my bed every night is silent, when not even a cricket sings, not a sound, not a frog trilling or a bat zooming through the air. For now all is quiet except my mind.

Of course surreptitious night creatures lurk outside my fragile cocoon. Opossums swing by their tails from maple branches, beavers gnaw rings in trees with a mouthful of sharp hatchets, red foxes skulk after sleeping geese and skunks slink in the shadows where white-footed mice tiptoe through tall grasses nibbling seeds, trying to stay out of harm's way. Flying squirrels deftly glide through the blackness seeking food. Once this curious little animal landed on my seed tray and silently chewed his dinner.

In a moment of perversity, I miss the eerie howling of the coyotes as they pack their way across the black cornfield stalking blind moles and skittering mice, hoping for the more filling meal a goose would provide. And I miss the owl's lonesome hoot deep in the woods behind my house. I imagine him swiveling his head almost full circle and piercing the night with round, knowing eyes looking for poor, beleaguered mice. It's been a long time since I was startled awake by the ear-splitting screams of sleeping chickens being plucked off the branch of a tree by a marauding raccoon family or jolted out of a deep slumber by a sudden unidentified thump in the dark only to lie awake breathlessly listening for another.

I do know a lion's roar is far scarier at night as, of course, are night crimes that terrorize our dreams.

Thinking about night, I'm reminded that the sounds of evening are quite different. Late yesterday at dusk when the last hint of daylight lingered after the sun had disappeared, I heard the soft evensong of a bird settling down in the spruce. A cricket launched his chirruping without stopping for breath and a pair of tree frogs rasped loudly to one another somewhere in the darkening woods. Swifts and nightjars swooped and twittered above the treetops scouring the air for high-flying insects and at the woods' edge the leaf litter rustled under some small hoof, paw or maybe a thrush poked for insects as he finished dinner. From the window of my imagination I saw a family of deer tiptoe out of the roadside thicket to graze on the still succulent green shoots. They often come to the cornfield at dusk.

Throughout this night of wakefulness my loving cat has kept me company—purring loudly in my ear as she nestles with me under the moon blanket. Her contentment is so noisy it may have drowned out the usual scratchings, thumpings and rustlings that make my heart thud and Rosie snores as she stretches across my feet. She raises her sleepy head to look at me, then flops down on her stuffed bear. Fully awake with little hope of sleeping, I don't feel lonely or troubled. In fact, I'm basking in peace knowing I can make up the loss of sleep in the morning if I want to.

My thoughts return to the mysteries of night. I believe our bodies grow and heal in the dark—cells rejuvenate during sleep. Meandering, I think about other happenings in the dark, like how flower buds swell, how plants seem taller in the morning and how some flowers bloom only at night. Exotic moths hungry for light bang their large-eyed wings against windows, the tooth fairy comes to leave her coin when we're asleep, Santa Claus drops down chimneys and ghosts visit at night. Canada geese migrate at night, their invisible regiment vees south as if pulled by a magnet. Where my imagination wanders in daylight, it flies in the dark and my thoughts tumble over one another. By now the moon has crossed over the sky window and a glittery star has taken its place. I measure the moon's progress, then the star's, then a milky cluster of stars as they move steadily westward with the rolling earth. Clouds of morning cross their paths and flow east across my small square of window, which has inspired hours of meditation. It's like an infinite movie screen. My eyelids have become heavy and my thoughts slow to a crawl just as dawn lights the sky window.

# October

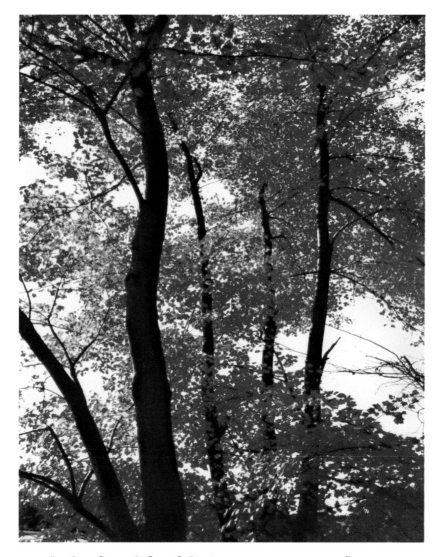

"I the fiery life of divine essence, am aflame
beyond the beauty of the meadows, I gleam
in the waters, and I burn in the sun, moon,
and stars…I awaken everything to life."

*Hildegard de Bingen*

# October Journal

## October 4

Dawn grayed the sky and cold rain splattered the skylight, blurring the windows and making it impossible to see out. Rosie spent the morning asleep, curled up like Wyeth's golden dog on the sofa bed. For a while I watched her side rise slowly, almost imperceptibly as she breathed. The rain, interspersed with patches of drizzle has lasted most of the day. I've neither walked nor accomplished much of anything except reverie. This afternoon I reminisced about my mother's sayings and how so many of them had to do with nature and wild creatures. I have no idea where she'd heard them, but she made them colorfully hers.

When my mother was pleasantly surprised she'd exclaim, "Lord, love a duck!" If something struck her as very good it was "the bee's knees, the cat's meow" or its pajamas. If someone didn't fit into her notion of how one should be, they were a "fish out of water" and if lacking material necessities, "poor as a church mouse." A person might be "smart as a fox, deaf as a fence post" or "dead as a doornail." If I clumsily knocked over a glass of milk, I was a "bull in a china shop" at which point she "took the bull by the horns" and curbed my errant behavior by "nipping it in the bud." My mother wasn't going to get caught "up a creek without a paddle" if humanly possible and if she were in such an unfortunate predicament, she hoped the misfortune slid off her "like water off a duck's back." This didn't happen often, but there was "no beating around the bush" where she was concerned and her impatience impelled her to drive like a "bat out of hell, straight as a crow flies" to her destination. Listening to these sayings with a child's literal ear, I wondered what was special about bee's knees. I imagined cats in pajamas and bats streaming out of some hot place. My mother never believed in herself enough to know how "right as rain" she was when she trusted her instincts and called upon the creatures.

## ❍ *October 6*

I was wakened suddenly at 4:00 A.M. by a shuddering wave of anxiety—not exactly a sense of foreboding, followed by smaller washes of fear rising out of some deep place strong enough to stop my breath. This morning I feel snappish. I don't know why. My life feels really good right now. I'm healthy, I'm photographing what I love, work is going well and I'm seeing friends and family often. Best of all I'm writing with more determination than ever. But the pressure to get going on my book idea and the daunting amount of work ahead seems to have brought me to another edge of my life where transition has crept up behind me and is pushing me into the unknown.

Jean Shinoda Bolen, author of *Close to the Bone*, reassures me that all the feelings I've experienced since learning I had breast cancer are normal and she writes, "So the next time you encounter fear, consider yourself lucky. This is where courage comes in. Usually we think that brave people have no fear. The truth is that they are intimate with fear." I am comforted.

Still, as the cancer-free years pass, too often I become immersed in daily minutiae or I sink into a bog of worry, spending too much time thinking about the life I have left and whether or not I'm living it well. Too easily I forget the preciousness of each day. When periodic clouds descend on me, I'm swamped with the knowledge that I really have no choice but to dance along a high wire where fear of a life-endangering disease, for the moment gone dormant, competes with a deep desire to attend to the moment at hand, and learn to let go.

Soul work may not be about self-pity but it's downright tiring. In the past seven years I've ridden enormous waves of feeling like a novice surfer and crashed to the depths of gritty terror, plunged into quagmires of shameful thoughts and found that self-discovery is a daunting task.

Just when I think I've bottomed out, just when I've thought it impossible to get up and out, I've discovered strengths I had no idea existed amidst all the messiness. Confidence builds little by little. I can make a book. With so much going so right for me now I can't afford to look so hard for meaning especially when it's slapping me in the face.

My mood has improved this afternoon after a morning connecting with clients who teach me as much as I do them. A long walk with Rosie, reading a good book and straightening up my desk have also helped. At lunchtime I visit with a friend who's had breast cancer and we explore the dark places, the intolerable feelings together until we finally poke fun at disease and death and laugh at ourselves. There lies the best tonic—laughter. I've decided I'm not in a pit, but making another shaky ascent into uncertainty and the possibility of failure—ancient bugaboos that have plagued me for a lifetime. I will make a book. Slowly I'm coming to realize life isn't static, can never be and I mustn't let moments of joy slip by unnoticed and I needn't evade moments of painful reflection. It's okay to be fully in either place.

## ⚬ *October 9*

Awaking too early this morning, I'm filled with contentment. A soft, purring cat licks my nose "good morning" and a sleepy golden dog laps my ear. If I'm careful not to crack an eye open I think both will give up trying to wake me. Through my lashes I see all eyes close and the three of us breathe deep breaths into sleep wrapped in happiness. Hazel, purring so passionately she chokes, rouses me again. Through the sky window the moon glows in the iris of a delft-blue sky like the chalky pupil of an eye before it inches toward the western horizon.

At lunchtime, Rosie and I take a quick walk around the bog. The maples are on fire—scarlet, orange and scalding yellow leaves dance like flames in the southerly breeze. I've noticed how their branches tend to grow skyward, yet their twigs and leaves are layered downward like an umbrella. I wonder if this is to better catch the sunlight. One spectacular tree leaves its own circle of sun beneath its yellow canopy.

Rosie trots just ahead of me, as always with a sweet grin on her face, her ears alert to small sounds rustling under fallen leaves. She stops to sniff at some invisible something, which proves uninteresting and with a snort, moves on ignoring the deer tracks in the sandy trail. I follow the tracks for a while until they disappear into the cranberry meadow. Along the roadsides and at the edges of the fields the rowdy succession of bloom that's filled wild places since April has passed in a rush of last-minute color that dazzles the eye. Purple asters compete with red blueberry bushes and milkweed hulls crack open letting their white parachutes go. Long before I come upon them, patches of fern give off a rich herbal aroma. They've turned all shades of pale green to light ochre and cinnamon and some have browned until their curled dry fronds crumble in my fingers. I'm astonished when a solitary and ragged monarch butterfly flutters by me rising higher and higher into the azure sky until it disappears. How will this tattered insect survive the long journey he has before him so late in the season?

## ⚬ *October 10*

It's late afternoon and I'm sitting at a picnic table under a stand of oak saplings growing at the edge of a bluff, which drops sharply to meet the incoming tide on the coast of Maine. To my right the sun is dropping behind a clutch of pines across an inlet. The tide inches its way up and over long flat, striated rocks until it lifts a bed of shiny sea grasses with a gentle nudge. They wave upright beneath the rising green water and the ocean reclaims its shore. We've settled on this campsite for our annual leaf-peeping and therapeutic-shopping weekend in Freeport. If I close my eyes I can smell the salt air and am lulled by the shooshing sound of small waves nipping at the base of the bluff. The only other sound is the "caw-caw" of crows across the inlet. Barry has taken the dogs for a walk.

Neither of us slept well last night, perhaps because we were both covered with dogs sharing our narrow camp beds, but this morning dawned with a brilliant sun in a cloudless sky and being on the coast has an ineffable healing capacity so we awoke in good moods. By afternoon a flotilla of giant white clouds sailed in from the east. When the sun poked out between the flying billows, maples and oaks and birches glistened with scarlet, orange, crimson and yellow radiance. At lunch we drove along Route One to Sheepscott where we found a picnic spot on the outskirts of this lovely village lying along the banks of a drowsy river. Sumac groves splashed with orange-red bordered the roadsides; both smooth and staghorn sumac flower heads are deep crimson. We ate our picnic in a sunny circle beneath the golden canopy of an ancient maple.

### October 11

I woke early to an unexpectedly brisk, clear morning (the forecast for today was dismal). Yet, as I write a blustery north wind is shoving large storm clouds across the sky. Patches of deep blue open between clouds to let in sudden shafts of light, which shower the leaves and mosses carpeting the woods around our camper. In a bit of a mood I get up before the others and dress for an early walk alone. I seem to need solitude more often than not these days, especially when traveling. I head for the shore and climb down on the rocks where the tide has begun to creep in along the crevices. At the shore's edge a tangle of wild rosebushes, barberry and squashberry bushes sparkle with glossy red fruits. Further down along the bluff a mountain ash leans precariously over the edge drooping with heavy clusters of orange berries. Seagulls warm and preen themselves on the flat rocks extending into the inlet. I walk out as far as I can to photograph them. The birds let me approach quite close before they rise in a swarm and fly out of range. When I move back they return. I've violated their circle of safety and should know better. Leaving the rocks and the birds I walk toward the woods bordering the tidal inlet and spot a great blue heron fishing in the shallows. He too flaps away when he sees me coming.

Bunches of ground-hugging wintergreen plants can scarcely keep secret their crimson berries nestled among their shiny leaves. Clumps of cinnamon and bracken ferns, still woodsy green, sway beside the trail end, which opens onto a meadow. The land we're camping on is part of a working farm and when I cut across the meadow, I startle a flock of sheep nuzzling the short grass. A small herd of Jersey heifers, looking like deer with large doey eyes and fawn-colored hides, graze in the corner of another pasture. I say "hi" to the group and the heifers turn to look at me with curiosity. When I was a child, we raised Jerseys on the farm and I remember being told their milk was creamier than that of any other cow. A large dollop of thick cream had to be scooped from the bottle before we could pour out a glass of milk. I hated the thick milk and the creamy mustaches it left around my mouth.

Unlike inland vegetation, the oaks and maples along the shore and in the woods are still summer green. Only a few have turned color. The farmer's garden is filled with morning glories, blue as a patch of sky. Pink cosmos and zinnias, all past their prime, put on a final show, while yellow daisies and purple asters bloom furiously in the chilled air.

I feel much better when I return to camp. Barry has cooked a special breakfast with forbidden pieces of crispy bacon, two easy-over eggs and toasted bagels. Both dogs are tied to nearby trees and whine piteously wanting to get closer to our hearty breakfast. When we're done and packed to go, we take the dogs for a walk around the same loop from which I've just returned. The sun flickers on every surface—on oak leaves, on asters and piles of little yellow mushrooms, which still hold the memory of last night's rain in glittery droplets. Pure white clouds have replaced the dark ones that passed through early this morning. The dogs sniff every clump of wet grass, every tree and shrub and cover twice the distance we do before we return to camp.

I lie back against the front seat of the camper as we sing down the highway toward home. The sky looks like an upside-down landscape of deep blue oceans, cloud mountains, streams and gray flat meadows; it's so big here, I'm reminded of Montana's sky. It takes my breath away to see the radiant foliage against the backdrop of enormous cloud banks and deep green of spruces and pine lit by an in-and-out sun. The two landscapes compete for glory in my eyes this afternoon as we whiz down the turnpike where the most brilliant colors line either side of the road. I groan at the missed photo opportunities, but finally I let go and allow myself to be spellbound by the riot of colors.

## *October 12*

This morning another sky full of clouds changes its persona by the minute. The clouds thin until they completely disintegrate and the sky window fills with pure blue. Through the front window the yellow-orange leaves of the old maple are drifting down around its craggy trunk and the viburnum has changed from dark green to burnished red. A flock of homely female house sparrows snatches breakfast at the window feeder and when they're finished they go for a splash in the birdbath. I've reconsidered my opinion of these unremarkable, ubiquitous and drab little brown birds. This morning they're enchanting and endearing as they go about their communal activities like a group of women enjoying each other's company; their chatter sounds like laughter to my ears. They're filled with playfulness when they bathe and chase one another out of the water into the branches of the viburnum and back again. Opening the door to let Rosie out startles the sparrows into a gust of wings and the ladies settle themselves out of harm's way deeper in the shrubbery. The males don't join in this morning ritual. They appear more sedate, even solitary, preferring to spend their time at quieter feeding stations.

The bird book tells me house sparrows roost together during the chilling fall and chillier winter nights, their numbers providing a huddle of warmth. When breeding season arrives in the spring, the flock breaks up into pairs competing fiercely for nesting sites. Today the entire flock gathers again at midday and this time with the males in attendance, the group chirps and scolds during the entire lunch hour.

## October 17

I'm surprised to find the cranberry meadow flooded this afternoon. The harvest has begun and machines beat the cranberries loose from their submerged stems until they rise to the surface and float in reddish-pink rafts on the black water. The water birds love this unexpected feast and a group of jabbering mallards swims through the mats of cranberries leaving little wakes as they go. A flock of six tiny sandpipers skims across the bog flashing their white wings over its red surface. They look like flying origami birds. More swamp maples have let go their foliage and Rosie and I slush through carpets of buttery yellow leaves. Oak trees having waited until the blazing spectacle of color put on by the maples has dimmed, don their claret, terra cotta, mauve and burnt-orange regalia and this afternoon their leaves, backlit by the setting sun, glisten and trace delicate patterns against the cerulean sky. On our way home Rosie and I dodge showers of acorns hurtling down on us.

## October 21

On our walk around the bog, Rosie and I came upon a small painted turtle who'd just crawled out of the flooded meadow, its carapace covered with splotches of bright green duckweed and dotted with cranberries. It clambered slowly into the tall grass and pushed toward the woods. I wondered if it knew it was decorated so. As we round the corner of the upper pond, the great blue heron is stalking. I stop to admire her focus, her steady concentration as she fishes, and wish I too could learn such pure meditation. Her homely face is utterly dignified, her stance elegant. Suddenly she spears a frog and gulps it down the length of her reedy, S-shaped gullet. I'd gag on such a bite. Hearing our approach the heron lifts herself with a grand whisper of wings up and out of the shallows and flaps low across the cranberry meadow to the edge of the lower pond. I'd have thought she'd flown south by now.

## October 28

I crack open my eyes at the sudden jangle of the alarm. On its way to California a large red moon hangs in the arms of a dead oak poking its branches into a vault of blue. I've decided the moon's face is that of a woman, a sad woman with eyes running with dark tears. Last night clouds streamed across the moon's face and still she shone with such brilliance, her light plunged into roadside thickets, into the forest and spread across the cornfield where three deer nibbled grass. A winter bite hardened the night air and through my open window I smelled moldering leaves and frostbitten flowers. As I settled down for the night, an airplane crossed the indigo sky, its twinkling wing lights dimmed by the moon's greater radiance. With her great orb fixed in my imagination, I took three deep breaths and closed my eyes for sleep. Suddenly I felt an odd sensation. My heart. Not only did I feel each beat, I actually heard it in this quiet night.

Slowly, steadily, my heart beat its own song. I've felt it pound crazily with anxiety and fear and sometimes I've even heard my pulse thump behind my ear, but this was different. The sound came from my chest. I'm filled with amazement at how this small organ pumps life through my body, blending its music with my breathing in and out until I finally I fall asleep.

I once thought October a dreary month, heading as it does into winter, but as this month ends I'm looking at the last gleaming maples, still gold and making their own sunlight as they stand among the leafless ones. Darkness comes earlier now that we've set our clocks back and the slant of late afternoon sun burnishes the oaks, some still dressed in crimson. Their branches are silhouetted against the bluest sky like skeins of lace. In the cornfield Canada geese spread out in a large congregation to glean seeds and bathe in the last rays of sunlight before rising with a noisy beat of wings and honking, to spend the night at the bog. As I write, a solitary oak leaf has landed on the sky window for a moment and rattles off in the breeze.

## ⌒ *October 31*

What must it be like to fly high in a downpour hatless, without goggles? A flock of starlings just flew with great speed over the sky window heading south. I don't envy them their wet journey this morning. The rain splatters against the roof and runs in rivulets down the windows making visibility impossible. The gutters drip a constant rhythm on this gray and dismal last day of October. Only a brave and bedraggled chickadee flies in for a seed before taking shelter in the hemlock.

## The Heron

She stands tall on a snag in the shallows—still
reflected in molasses water among skeleton trees and brittle reeds.

Her beak scissors open, then closes.
She gasps, not for air, but in pain; her shoulder is awkwardly bent.

She's hurt and hanging on, cannot give in,
cannot let her stilt legs fold and fall at last into the mirror.

Her steady meditation stiffens with pain in the end.
She's indifferent to my presence. I cannot help. I tell her goodbye.

When I return, she's gone, sunk into the murky water
or flown away. I wish for her flight, but know otherwise.

I know I'll see her—or another—stand so still or strut with grace
stalking minnows among lily pads, piercing quiet pools with her golden eye.

I'll be there when she spears a gleaming fish. I know
I'll watch her spread her great blue wings; with hardly a whisper they'll lift her gently
onto the wind and with slow and measured beats, she'll fly away.

# Anniversary

October is the anniversary of my mother's death. Her death was sudden and it devastated our family. Each of us knew her in our special way and each of us grieved losing her in our own way. My family never recovered losing its center and reason for gathering together. As the oldest, even I couldn't fill my mother's shoes and perhaps I didn't feel up to it. Each of us went our separate ways, even moved far away.

After weeks of pining for my mother—there was so much I wished I'd told her—I put her away in a deep recess of my heart and tried to fill the space left by her absence. The first holidays without her were especially sad for me. My family made a last heroic effort to celebrate the final Christmas we'd all have together.

Six months later I discovered a lump in my breast and my mourning came to an abrupt end as I struggled to cope with my fear and stumbled through the months of treatment. I desperately needed my mother; I needed her soothing. And yet, at the same time, I was grateful she wasn't there to witness me having to deal with what was her own worst nightmare—cancer.

# *October Death—1992*

Beside a warming fire you chatted over tea.
It was three weeks until your birthday
and the view from your window was browned
by a frost creeping across the pasture.

I watched you suddenly clutch your head
and crumple in your chair with the worst
in a lifetime of headaches. Silence
broken only by your labored breath
wrapped around you;
you never opened your eyes,
you never spoke again.

In the hospital your strong heart throbbed
flooding your head and they offered
machines to pump you back to life
if we wanted we could hang on to you
a while longer—knowing it was your nightmare;
frantic efforts to keep you stopped.
You lay alone, straining to breathe, your life
—a blip on a screen—ticked slowly irrevocably away.
I smoothed your matted hair. I wanted you to hear how much I loved you;
I wanted you to know you could go; we'd be all right.
Then, I'm certain I felt in my hand
the faintest movement of your fingers
and you were gone.

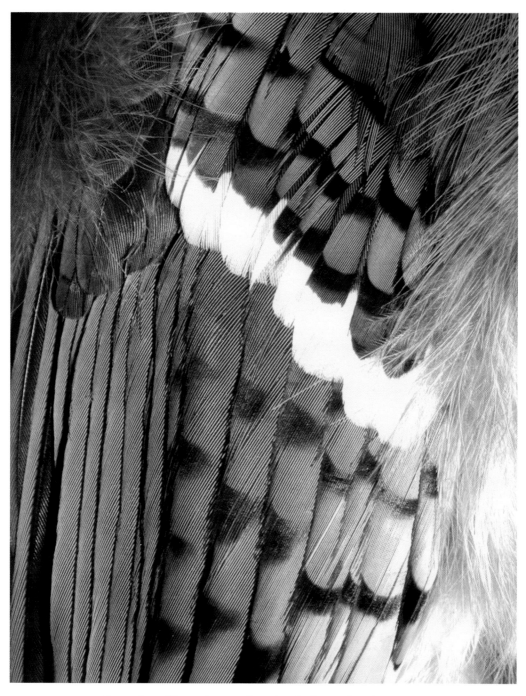

"To the illuminated mind the whole
world burns and sparkles with light."
*Ralph Waldo Emerson*

# The Hemlock

Just outside my office window a very old hemlock grows tall enough to dwarf the house and shelter it from the north wind. Waiting for winter, I look out my window and imagine its branches thick with dark green needles bent earthward laden with snow. I know how they'll pop up when a gust of wind topples their load sending glittery dust into the frigid air. Sheltering close to the trunk and hidden behind the hemlock's drooping arms dark-eyed juncos, nuthatches, chickadees and titmice flit and squirrels scold. My reverie is interrupted by a brilliant cardinal perched like royalty high in the hemlock watching over his mate while she takes her turn at the seed tray below. Surely, he knows how startlingly handsome he is.

When the sun slouches toward the horizon leaving the air chilled, I imagine the cardinal pair finding shelter in the crook of a branch where they'll huddle together and dream away the frigid night. Where do the chickadees go with their feathers plumped against the cold like down jackets? How does it feel to be a puffed up chickadee waiting through the long night for daylight and the warmth of the sun? If they're lucky, they find abandoned woodpecker holes and other nooks to shelter out of the wind.

One summer I dragged an old lawn chair inside the circle of the hemlock's floppy branches. Here I felt safely cocooned, invisible to the outside world. Only the chipmunks and a red squirrel noisily protested the invasion of their haven. I sat where the sun dappled the floor near the craggy trunk, a thick carpet of brown needles and tiny cones at my feet, and was reminded of the feeling I'd had as a child when I'd been scolded. I'd stamped away from home and gone to the woods where I found a cozy spot to make myself a hideout of fir branches shaped like a lean-to. I'd soften the ground with armfuls of pine needles and moss until it felt like a nest where I could sit and sulk until my attention was inevitably captured by a chipmunk shuffling around in the leaves searching for his stash of seeds or a curious titmouse alighting on a nearby sapling to check me out. It seems I've made nests all my life wherever I've found myself.

Two Octobers ago I was working in my office when I heard the dogs begin to bark with an unusual urgency. Glancing out of my open window, a large, black bear stood under the branches of the hemlock. I couldn't believe my eyes. Rosie and Gus were going crazy, but the bear appeared confident their whining and barking wasn't a threat. He ambled out from under the tree and attacked a large feeder hanging off a pole. Sunflower seeds sprayed all over his head and muzzle until finally it crashed to the ground. The bear lapped up the seeds and mauled the feeder for more, then lifted his head to sniff the air.

To get a better look, I'd leaned further out the window, too close for his liking and the bear shot me a look of disdain before lumbering to the edge of the woods at the back of the yard. Here he stopped beside another feeder filled to the brim with seed. Throwing caution to the wind he helped himself. By the time he'd crushed this feeder, I'd had time to grab my camera and ran out the back door where, safe behind the garden fence, I tried to capture him on film. My hands shook so much from excitement that in the end the results were blurred and disappointing. Talking to him from behind the fence seemed not to disturb his feasting and when he'd finished he began to tour the perimeter of the yard looking for more treats—at this point I wondered if he might not enjoy me as his main course. With as much ferocity as I could muster, I shouted, "Go home, bear!"

He looked at me and snuffed, then turned and disappeared into the woods. The bear returned once the next night. I could barely make out his dark form, but I heard the rattling of feeders being knocked down and muffled grunts as he munched sunflower seeds. After this visit, he never returned. The local newspaper made serious note of black bear sightings in yards all over Carlisle. I never told anyone of my visitor fearing he'd come to harm.

My imagination flows around the hemlock outside my window. I wonder what it's seen, what history it's witnessed. Has it watched children grow up in this house as the old elm watched me so long ago? And was the hemlock here before the house was built fifty years ago? Nestled as my house is in the arms of the hemlock, I share its shelter with so many creatures whose comings and goings I can observe from my window and whose company I treasure.

# November

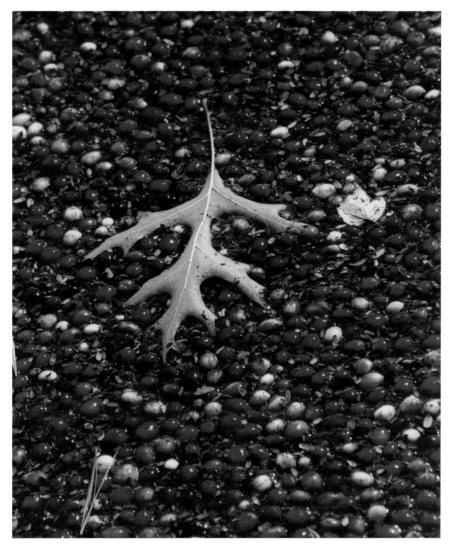

"The first peace, which is the most important, is that which courses within the souls of people when they realize their relationship, their oneness, with the Universe and all its powers, and then they realize that at the center of the Universe dwells the Great Spirit, and that this center is really everywhere, it is within each of us."

*Black Elk*

# November Journal

*November 3*

This morning as Rosie and I entered the woods at the edge of the pond, a small bird accompanied us along the path, flitting from branch to bush to twig to bramble just at eye level and just a step ahead of me. His small size and coloring suggested a chestnut-sided warbler, but they don't hang around this far north so late in the fall; maybe he was a yellow-rumped warbler, who does over-winter here. My little friend had a very yellow head, especially noticeable when flying into a shaft of sunlight. Could he be a blackpoll warbler in fall plumage? Obviously I know precious little about warblers. I do know this little bird seemed to be deliberately leading me and I followed him until the path became too difficult for me to continue. The little bird disappeared into a thicket.

Looking up at a white wintry sun veiled by motionless, thin diaphanous clouds, I think of the gift the warbler has given me; a summer bird flying into winter, connecting with another creature along the way. I can barely make out the whisper of my shadow in the pale blue light and Rosie and I turn for home. I've noticed that most of the red winterberries have been picked from the thicket of shrubs growing in a marshy patch beside the road. They hang from soft gray twigs like bright scarlet beads. Damn! I'd been waiting for just the right time to pick them for Christmas decorating. Just a few twigs of winterberry commands an exorbitant price at the garden shop and when I saw these little bunches, I thought smugly of all the free berries I'd collect at home by the bog. Foolish me.

Studying nature by reading and daily observation has raised questions, answered some, peaked my imagination and nourished me. I'm comforted by my growing familiarity with my place in the small patch of nature I inhabit. I fit in here with a purpose no matter what may come. As long as I'm aware of what's around me at any given instant, I'm sure to find sacred moments in even the most mundane circumstances, the smallest touch, the smell of my granddaughter when I kiss her behind her ear and make her giggle. A fleeting thought, a whiff of pine pitch, a sudden glimpse of deer or being led through the woods by a tiny bird are moments I treasure.

## November 6

A day forecasted to be dreary and full of mist has been transformed by the wind and copious sunshine so Rosie and I take a quick turn around the bog this morning. The heron doggedly persists in fishing for the last minnows and frogs that have yet to burrow into the bottom muck of the pond. Heading nowhere in particular, a flock of crows plays with the brisk wind high over the cranberry meadow. They topple and coast, tip and dive and then climb into the sky in an elegant dance. I've never seen this lighter side of dark and raucous crows; I could almost like them for this trait. I'm convinced I'd curl up in a maudlin ball of self-pity unless the silly side of life, mine in particular, didn't whack me on the side of the head now and again and make me laugh and want to play.

Driving down the highway after visiting with a friend in Cambridge, my attention veers off the road with a swarm of starlings who rise from a tree like a school of sparkling minnows. With a profusion of wings, they tilt, a single flying organism, dipping and bending against a cloudless, azure sky, until all at once the throng drops into a bare tree.

Late this afternoon a lovely, solitary song floated through the porch window. I thought it might be a winter wren, a species of wren I'd never seen before, but now I wonder if this diminutive bird isn't a male Carolina wren who not only sings all year long, but is able to sing up to forty versions of his song. Is it only male wrens who sing?

It's getting colder. The ponds are covered with a thin layer of ice and the ground has hardened with frost. More and more birds have returned to the feeding stations located all around my house. I've discovered that while these birds dine regularly here, most of their meals are found in the wild, which makes me think that for them, grabbing a meal at my house is like stopping at McDonald's for fast food when a gourmet restaurant is just around the corner. I still catch myself wondering what the birds say to one another and if two different species have found ways to communicate with one another—maybe with universal sign language.

Bare of leaves, the trees are now filled with tight-fisted buds. Only a few curled and brown oak leaves cling to naked branches and crackle with the slightest breath. A stiffer wind drags the clingers off and sets them sailing into the steely sky before hurling them rattling to the ground. The tops of evergreens are loaded with cones of all shapes and sizes. I don't recall seeing cones in such abundance in past years, but maybe I didn't notice. They too are flung to the ground with the wind and I collect baskets of pine cones to burn in the fireplace or to just inhale their woodsy aroma.

## ⌒ *November 13*

Today the November air is perfectly cold. The sky is hung with thick gray clouds moving slowly eastward until eventually a dime-sized sun thrusts itself out from behind the flowing clouds and a patch of blue opens up like a welcome gift. Rosie bounces ahead of me down the path to the pond. There's a bounce in my step too as I work to keep up with her. Once again the heron is stalking the ditches. When we disturb her concentration, she rises out of the ditch and lands in another further along the dike. Each time Rosie and I approach, we violate her circle of safely and the large bird lifts up and flaps quietly away, and each time I'm awed by her grace and my encounter with her.

The banks of the pond are spiked with stalks of goldenrod, joe-pie weed, all long gone to seed and brown grasses known as weeds in my still limited lexicon of wild flora. Chet Raymo, author of *Natural Prayers*, reframes for me the entire meaning of weed. Like so many others I've been guilty of relegating many wildflowers to the weed family, a category of noxious, unseemly and wildly prolific plants, which grow where few others dare and where the less hardy can't survive.

Mr. Raymo believes there's not much difference between ubiquitous, opportunistic and pesky flora and the human species. Like weeds we've overrun the habitats of other species, even our own, elbowing out the least hardy until we've attained the highest status on the food chain and populated ourselves in impossible lands. We've learned to survive natural disasters, build our homes in inhospitable deserts, shores and mountaintops; we've bent the natural world as much as is possible to suit our needs. Until now we've been relatively successful in this disastrous endeavor. And like weeds, we humans are prolific and ubiquitous and consume the greatest amount of the world's resources.

I think it's not too much of a stretch to cast ourselves in the category of weeds. With cocky arrogance we assume the earth will forever give up her endless riches if only we dig deep enough or lay bare wider swaths of landscape or use our considerable ingenuity to manipulate nature's essential makeup. We're confident she can absorb our profuse waste; that rivers and oceans will eventually wash us clean and that dirty air will pollute someone else's neighborhood. While we haven't exactly moved mountains Old Testament–style, we've dug holes through them and cut their tops off. I'd think even the hardiest weeds would succumb and fall victim to their own promiscuous prolificity, but we poison them, mow them down, dig them up and when we're sure we're rid of them, they surprise us in the spring. A dandelion pops up and winks at us.

I love the wild morning glory that spreads her vines into inconvenient places; with secret glee I cheer the golden dandelion blossoms infesting my neighbor's sterile lawn as well as my own weed-filled greensward. Their faces are full of spring's first warmth, their spent heads let loose drifts of seeds hung from silky filaments—a million prisms brimming with rainbows. Now I pay attention to milkweed whose gentle perfume and sweet nectar entice monarch butterflies to stay and lay their eggs. I gather bouquets of Queen Anne's lace and goldenrod to decorate my house. In summer when the banks of the ditches and bog ponds are scraped clean of weeds, I know they'll find a way to return because they know their place in nature's scheme and while they may overrun our human habitat, unlike human weeds, they'll give themselves up to nature's plan if asked to make room for another species to grow. And so I admire their resourcefulness, their courage. Rosie and I pass the upper bog pond rimmed with a forest of dried weed stalks still holding the memory of last summer in their empty seed heads and the promise of another season.

Rounding the corner of the pond a lone redwing blackbird perches high up in the dead pine singing his "cooleege" song. He's definitely not supposed to be here this late in the fall. In fact by the end of August most of his species have left the bog and gone south. I wonder why he stays and why the heron still lingers on in the deepening cold. Rosie and I scuttle up a flurry of little brown sparrows whose only sound is a whoosh of wings. The clouds have moved off and the afternoon light is mysterious, perfect for thinking about magical things like weeds and tardy migrants. Above us the low sun gilds the belly of a red-tailed hawk riding a thermal updraft high in the winter-blue sky.

## November 21

Except for the bare trees today is so balmy it feels like a day in early April. A pair of bluebirds sits on the branch of a tree at the edge of the cornfield surveying the brown landscape. Bluebirds often stay through the winter but they never come to the feeding stations. Uncharacteristically silent, a mockingbird hops through the roadside thicket leading me toward the bog. In an oak sapling a pine warbler no longer hidden by foliage sits bobbing his tail up and down. He's delicately small—grayish with light wing bars and sports a sharp beak. I'm still having a hard time figuring out who's who in the warbler family, especially since these tiny birds change their plumage in the fall and immature birds have yet to don adult garb.

Most surprising today was passing a young buck standing in the cornfield when I drove to town. I stopped the car to stare at him and he stared right back at me before stepping deliberately across the rough field. The shorn cornstalks look like a stubbly beard poking out of the earth's dark skin.

## November 22

Late this afternoon I walked beside my long shadow in the slanting sunlight until rounding a corner down at the bog, it jumped up in front of me—taller than I've ever wished to be. Turning another corner, my shadow disappeared and a thin scrim of clouds blurred the contours of the sun settling into the horizon. I didn't see my shadow again. Rosie and I headed home under a pale, cold sky, now turning bluer. Wisps of pink clouds hung along the horizon like flowing ribbons. My heart lifts to join a flight of Canada geese honking overhead. I wonder what it would be like to fly with so many friends and family. I'm quite sure the goose families I made friends with this spring are up there—the young ones loving the sensation of air beneath their wings and the music of their companions.

Lately I've been thinking about solitude. I'm reminded of a quote from *The Desert Year*, by Joseph Wood Krutch. "To have passed through life and never experienced solitude is to never have known oneself. To have never known oneself is to have never known anyone." In the past several years I've not only learned to appreciate solitude more, but find it's become crucial to my well-being. Growing older and perhaps a little wiser has dramatically changed my capacity for being alone. Not so long ago I was driven to fill the silence around me with busyness and with people, but curiously, none of this activity mitigated the loneliness I felt. Being alone with myself used to be painfully distressing. In brief moments of clarity—those rare glimpses of reality—it occurred to me that I was perfectly alone when I came into this life and will be again when I leave it. What I do in between is up to me and has little to do with the presence or absence of others. A frightening thought. Being quiet in that place where self-discovery is nourished takes a bit of courage and doing nothing takes practice.

Doing nothing has always meant something wasn't getting done that should be done. It meant inattention and laziness, it meant loosening the vigilance necessary to prevent the untidiness of life from creeping in and taking over my days and it meant something infinitely more terrifying and impossible—being quiet, being alone and being with myself. Doing nothing now requires a new definition. These days I take a large gulp of breath before diving deep into the bottom of my soul—down through restless thoughts and rumbling emotions, down past illusions and contradictions, ambivalence, meanness and the fear of what I might still discover. More often than not I land with a thunk and all the messiness tumbles around me. The miracle is, I'm still breathing.

Occasionally, when I rise above the mess, I see myself in my life with a perspective I've never before experienced. It's then I'm less terrorized by the shadowy self that lurks behind the surface noise and begin to learn to live with uncertainties impossible to resolve. Most compelling for me is the knowledge that I'm flawed and perfect all at the same time. So much time has been wasted aspiring to perfection or striving to control its illusion. It's taken an inordinate amount of effort to deny or disguise shameful weaknesses. Domesticating these hardwired parts of me hasn't been easy and I've only just begun to relax the struggle. Doing nothing now means not having to be busy and it means not letting myself be overcome by insidious restless thoughts and it means knowing what I'm doing when I'm in the midst of doing it.

The capacity to be with myself is but one consequence of learning to be still. Once in a while I've been able to quiet my thoughts long enough to experience a sense of peace. Something happens inside, which allows me to hear a whispering inner voice—my own. It soothes me and tells me all's well—at least for the moment. My legs won't bend to the lotus position to meditate. In fact, sitting doesn't work well for me. Such interludes are most likely to occur when I walk in nature. Trekking around the bog, strolling through the woods and across fields are walking meditations. I count my breaths and step mindfully so I can feel the ground beneath my feet. Peace spreads over me when I gaze at the blueness of the sky or lie with Rosie and Patches snuggled close. Standing very still to spy on a chickadee or a dragonfly through the lens of my camera or my own eye lets the moment's sensations fill my mind.

Solitude, being alone and stilling my mind long enough to listen to my voice and the voices of nature, has become a gift. I hear the voices more clearly: The sound of wings, of paddling in water, the songs of the wind—all the voices of the earth around me are constantly in the background of my awareness and more often than not, in the foreground.

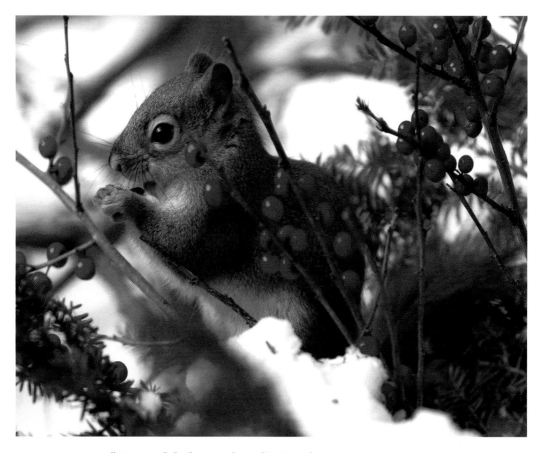

"On cold days, the divine haunts
the exhalations of squirrels
whose breath hovers
starch-white as tiny souls."

*Diane Ackerman*

# Becoming a Wise Woman

Somewhere in your mid-forties, if you paid attention to your life, you may have accumulated enough experiences to have gained a little wisdom. This is mostly because you've made so many mistakes so many times you finally get it and stop repeating them—maybe. A wise woman has learned to cherish her mind. She reads, listens and challenges her mind with new information, new ways of thinking, new experiences. She learns to form opinions of her own that are worth listening to. The fact is she's an avid student, hungry for all life can teach her, and she's confident that she can learn anything she puts her mind to. A wise woman hones skills, first by learning to listen more carefully; she listens to her own voice, then to her body and finally, making efforts to suspend judgment, to other voices. A wise woman is stronger than ever and softer at the same time. She moves furniture and cuddles.

A wise woman likes herself better than she did when she was twenty or thirty and it may take time before she can really accept herself—sometimes not until the ripe age of sixty. She knows she has blemishes, large ones, both physical and spiritual, but she's in the process of accepting these with a touch more grace. Though she cares for her body, she often bemoans the steady encroachment of wrinkles and sagging flesh. Even so, she glimpses the vital woman she really is when she looks at the truth in the mirror and can forgive herself for aging, for the lines of laughter creasing her eyes. Speaking of laughter, it tends to burst out of her more frequently because she's gotten better at appreciating the silly side of life. Yet, in spite of this, two sad-lines have carved themselves deep between her brows and tears come easier now that she doesn't need to hide them. It's possible she may become more beautiful with age—at least in her mind?

A wise woman also knows if she gives up just one scrap of her vitality she'll become invisible like other old ladies who do. She gets noticed because she likes to smile when there are no smiles in sight—at the grocery store, the bank, she smiles. She dares to catch a stranger's eye, grin and walk on by. Sometimes these moments of speechless connection are precious. Age has loosened her tongue, but she knows when to soften her words, to still them and when to set them free. Mostly she says what she thinks. She tries to be kinder than she used to be.

Shaking hands with her mortality has brought her wisdom. She's felt the fear and the loneliness that come with this inevitable knowledge. A wise woman has a special place for these thoughts. They don't hide in the recesses of her mind, nor do they rule her days. They lie quietly in her soul. Time is important to a wise woman because she knows how inexorably it moves forward and she's learning to care less whether or not she can keep up with it so long as she lives in it moment to moment.

Becoming a wise woman means shedding many old prohibitions, outdated rules and all the old voices absorbed long ago, which only served to stunt her being. Ridding herself of the old voices, the old ways hasn't been accomplished without painful effort and each step along the way, she's wondered if the letting go was the right thing to do. The old ways had their usefulness in her life and she understands why she's hung onto them for so long. Being gentle with herself, she accepts being a slow learner. Most of all a wise woman has become less fearful of her nakedness: she recalls most of her shameful detours and forgives the stupidity or stubbornness that drove her to stumble—all those mistakes she might have had control over—and let go of those she didn't. She never wants to go back and repeat her history. As she is now is okay. She knows she's always in the process of becoming more of whom she's become.

This woman on her way to becoming wise is running out of steam and wants to take a nap. She's feeling disappointed and a wee bit sorry for herself—she can do that too—because her husband hasn't listened to her and once again forgot how important it would have been if he'd remembered to send her flowers today.

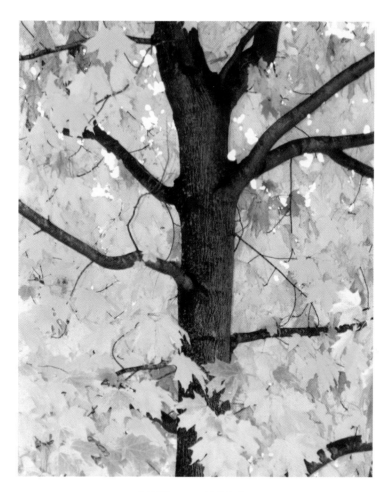

## When I Die

When I die
plant a tree close to me.
Hemlock, holly, buckthorn, oak—
it will not matter which
when I seep through the earth
like slow rain sipped by roots
I'll rise
skyward, pulled into branches, into twigs.
I'll feed unfolding leaves, I'll flower,
fruit and fill with seed.
I'll transpire
and with each green and glorious exhalation
I'll become
the air you breathe.

# December

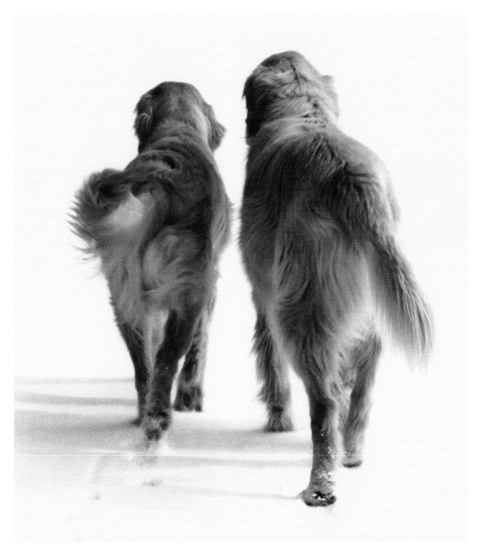

"Ask the animals and they will teach
you."

*Job 7–10*

# December Journal

### *December 1*

After the rain stopped, the sky has spat out enough snowflakes to sprinkle the ground. Rosie and I make our way to the bog and into the woods. An icy northwest wind messes with the heavy gray clouds still clotting the leaden sky. Clumps of furry green mosses brighten the crevices of granite rocks strewn throughout the forest and gray and orange lichens cling in soft rosettes to their hard, cold surfaces. I think these large and small boulders were dropped in the wake of receding glaciers eons ago. Brittle stalks of goldenrod, mullein and joe-pie weed are limned with snow and thickets of pine seedlings and hemlock boughs are covered with a light mantle of white dust and it all looks magical. Walking is particularly peaceful without the usual company of strident crows and blue jays that are curiously silent. Rosie and I stop suddenly when a doe steps tentatively across the path ahead of us and melts into the brambly thicket—the gift of a chance encounter doesn't escape me.

A mat of clouds covering the sky from horizon to horizon has me thinking about clouds—how they darken, blur or obliterate the sun; how clouds portend bad, even dangerous weather. How they fling down pellets of ice, scatter flakes of snow, and how they can fill the air with mist, drop rain or deluge the earth with water. Clouds are mercurial. They fly and sail with abandon, they're blown into white puffy shapes filling a blue canvas and the imagination. They climb into the sky suddenly or melt in the sun, but most amazing is how clouds grasp the last rays of sunlight and are transformed into breathtaking ribbons of molten color. I've come to love a sky full of clouds as much as I do a bowlful of blue or a pulsing sun.

My meditation turns to other discoveries; new loves found in the past year: I've learned to appreciate weeds as wildflowers. I'm captivated by a homely grasshopper as much as a monarch butterfly, a mole as much as a deer or even an elephant—all creatures great and small, plain and lovely, except for a select few, like snakes who have yet to convince me of their lovableness, much as I may appreciate their usefulness in nature's web. Practicing mindfulness and honing observation skills has given my world a wider perspective and now I've begun to "see clouds from both sides." Still, I have a ways to go—I don't love everything or everybody equally as I might, and some not at all. This may always be so, but perhaps my capacity to love will continue to develop as I watch and listen and understand more.

## December 9

It's a cold, cold day for a walk and I've decided to wait until late afternoon when the sun will have taken the edge off the sharp air. Down at the bog the lowering sun pours a stream of molten gold over the thickening ice across the pond and leaves puddles of light on the woods trail where the last oak leaves crackle under my feet. Walking on quiet, moccasin feet isn't possible this afternoon. The sky cradles bunches of swollen white clouds, which look as if they might loosen a shower of snow any minute. The wind has picked up and whooshes through the tops of the pines unhitching clusters of cones and flinging them to the ground. The trees creak and sing with each gust. Even the pond sings its eerie medley of rumbles as the ice contracts. Barry says he can tell the thickness of the ice just by looking at the web of hairline cracks, which appear with each groan. I'm not sure I believe him enough to test his hypothesis by walking on it.

The geese and crows stay close to the ground this afternoon. The heron fishes in the shelter of the cove in the upper pond. Now more than ever I'm worried he won't survive the winter, especially when the ditches are freezing over and the fish and frogs have gone under the muck. When Rosie and I approach the young heron spreads his wings and flies across the frozen bog meadow with a harsh call of irritation, which reminds me of the cranking sound when winding our grandfather clock. There was a time I dismissed herons as ugly, gawky birds. Rosie and I walk quickly toward home with the wind at our backs.

## December 11

After a night of snuggling with Rosie and Patches and a string of forgettable dreams, I awoke late. Dressed for the cold, Rosie and I are off to the bog. A small sun, the size of a dime, warms the air slightly, but just as we reach the bog a thin bank of clouds creeps in from the west and shrouds the sun. The breeze picks up enough to tumble some oak leaves, which follow us along the trail to the pond.

I've been thinking about Christmas and how only a few years ago after my mother died, I struggled to enter into the spirit of the holiday with the same enthusiasm I'd had for so many years before. I've learned to let go of most of what I loved about Christmas as my family has moved far away. Our family gatherings were special, the festivity, the excitement and anticipation of Christmas caught me up in a whirl of activity and heightened emotion. Our holiday began at Thanksgiving and lasted through New Year's.

For years my mother filled the holidays with her childlike spirit, and this she passed on to me. I'm not sure if other family members got so carried away. As the years passed and my mother became more frail, Christmas lost its magic for her. She crabbed about having to wrap a room full of presents and abdicated her role of Christmas fairy, delegating to others what she'd always loved to be in charge of. She began to dread the holidays and couldn't wait until they were over. Yet, her legacy infused my imagination and I ignored the wet blanket she threw over the festivities in her last years.

These days I've let go of beloved traditions I once thought I couldn't live without. I've reinvented this holiday by finding new ways to celebrate it and although the magic has dimmed a little, I still find pleasure in gathering with whoever is available, even if I have to travel a distance to do so. I'm still excited to find or make gifts for those I love and to decorate my house, filling it with greens and the aroma of pine.

## December 13

For some time now I've wondered why I haven't seen cottontail rabbits around my neighborhood. A few years ago they were hopping across the lawn or trying to squeeze under the vegetable garden fence. I loved seeing the little ones scampering out of their nest under the viburnum.

Recently I read an article in a regional nature magazine about rabbits. I was disturbed to learn that the two species of cottontails in New England are becoming extinct—the New England cottontail and the eastern cottontail. Apparently both species like to forage in fields and meadows and prefer to raise their young in the safety of thickets, bramble and scrub. Once so plentiful in my neighborhood, this type of habitat is disappearing at a frightening rate. Rampant development has cleared the fallow fields, meadows and thickets. Sweet clovers and grasses don't grow in the forest and nothing is particularly edible in the sterile lawns carpeting developed land. Rabbits are scared of humans and are easy prey to a burgeoning population of cats and dogs. How sad to think these Peter Rabbits of my childhood might soon be a dear memory.

## December 17

It's balmy today like it might be at the tail end of March. Rain pinged on the sky window all night and into the morning, then stopped long enough for us to chance a walk.

The leaf litter covering the woods trail is sodden and my feet make barely a sound as I walk past the shadows where small patches of ice still linger. A few Canada geese preen and converse softly with one another in the shallows where the ice has melted. I say "hello" and walk on by not wishing to disturb their peaceful gathering. Suddenly I'm startled by an up-rushing of equally startled mallards that have hidden in the shade of a ditch. Ten of them settle onto a safer patch of water.

Across the upper pond a tall, dead pine tree lifts bare dark branches into the gray sky above an evergreen crown of lesser trees. It has me thinking about a tree's life span. Why did this healthy specimen die? What shortened its life? There are obvious explanations—insect predation, disease attacking from within and without, age, storm damage and human interference.

Still standing tall, the old pine's naked branches provide a lookout for crows and hawks. Now and again I've seen a great blue heron perch in the tree to scan the pond below. Its trunk is home to nuthatches, chickadees and other creatures. Insects feed on its rotting core and woodpeckers feed on them. Finally when it's scoured bare, hollowed out and brittle, the wind or a snowfall will knock the skeleton tree to the ground where it becomes a shelter for mice and rabbits, until eventually it melts into the earth. Then one day, the seed it sowed before it died, coils out of the soil near its fallen parent.

The question is, does a tree really die or does its energy merely change form— giving its own life to bring life to others? I think I'm not so different from the tree since I too, am subject to the same predations and natural disasters. But when it's time I'm stripped to my core, I want to believe I'll give life back to the earth like the tree has. This line of thinking sends me into the forest where I hug the nearest live pine. Well, it's the only way to see clear to its top and the sky. The rough trunk feels good in my arms and I'm especially glad to be alive in this moment. Rosie and I hurry out of the woods and home just as rain begins to dribble out of the sky.

## ∿ December 19

Once again the bog pond is iced over and its surface, rippled by the big winds of a day ago, has been blown into frozen wavelets. A few geese sun themselves on the gravel path beside the shore and slide onto the ice when Rosie and I approach. A huge pulsing sun with a nimbus of light radiating around it warms my face.

At home the chickadees, dark-eyed juncos and woodpeckers crowd around the suet cakes I've put out for them. Taking a break from writing to watch the birds out my office window, something catches my eye just beyond the hemlock. A beautiful doe moves out of the shelter of the tree to stand under the bird feeders. For a moment she looks up at me in the window, then bends her head to nibble at the fallen seeds. Her ears are large and oval and rimmed with an extra layer of winter fur. Her eyes appear luminously black and as shiny as her nose, which begins to twitch just before she shambles off behind the house and out of sight. I turn off the computer, get in my car and head to Agway to buy deer food and a feeding trough as well as a salt block, which I'll place beside the thicket at the edge of the woods. And hope.

## ∿ December 22

I'm reading last year's journal entry for this date. An enormous full moon had risen in the southeastern sky and seemed larger and more brilliant than usual due to some astronomical confluence of heavenly events. This moon marked the winter solstice and was the last full moon of the century, which at the time was an awesome thought. The moon had made me smile and I wrote, "I honestly never thought six years ago I'd be here to witness the turn of the century. I wonder if others like me feel this way in this last month of 1999. In a way the first day of the new year is just another day, but I feel there's something momentous going to happen to me in the coming new year as I anticipate the birth of a grand daughter and begin to feel more comfortable in my skin and in my world. Life is exciting me more than ever it has in the past."

I feel much the same on the eve of another new year. This Christmas I'll share with Ilaria, whose presence in my life has rekindled all the playfulness I once felt. She's given me gift upon gift with her smiles and gurgles.

## December 29

Christmas Eve and the next day were filled with happiness because I spent much of the time with my grandbaby, who now reaches for me and laughs. I'm filled with my own giggles as Ilaria squinches up her eyes and pushes her little face toward Rosie, who obliges by licking the baby's face and fiercely wagging her tail. Christmas day was much like last year—bitterly cold with a strong wind that put the wind-chill factor below zero, I think. The wind lasted into the following day and I didn't walk.

Though it's tolerable, today is very cold. The wind has calmed down and Rosie and I are off to the bog. The cranberry meadow has been flooded to protect the tiny cranberry shrubs from this intense cold and the ice is slick enough for skating. Sometimes the pond is covered with black ice so clear I can see turtles moving slowly through the bottom weeds—it's a scene of suspended animation with still green stems reaching up to the thick glassy surface. The ice on the pond isn't clear now, but the frozen wavelets have smoothed out. Crows are nowhere to be seen and must be shouldering together deep in the woods to keep warm.

At home I've been especially careful to replenish all the feeders with seed and suet cakes. A flock of doves pecks at the ground for dropped seed and are joined by a couple of juncos. As I look out my window into the failing light, I'm sure I hear a robin calling. Is that possible?

## December 31

This last day of a memorable year is a lovely one filled with snow. It fell heavily all through the night and this morning the evergreen branches are draped in crystalline white. In fact the entire landscape is white until I look up into a cloudless, deep blue sky. Yesterday afternoon when the snow began, all the little creatures took cover and no one came back to the feeders for the rest of the day.

The new snowfall inspires me to get out of bed much earlier than is my habit and I can't wait to get outside to make first footprints. I dress quickly and

haphazardly. With my nightgown hitched up under a coat and tall boots on my bare feet, I grab my camera and wade through the
deep snow in the backyard to make tracks even before the dogs have a chance. After a while the sun travels around to the front of the house where the feeders are closest to the porch windows. I set up my camera and spend the rest of the morning photographing unsuspecting juncos, titmice, sparrows and chickadees in the warmth of the porch lit by a gleaming sun. I may have captured a wary blue jay as he flashed his Bermuda blue wing feathers. The resident pairs of cardinals look particularly splendid this morning perched in the green spruce branches still covered with snow.

Near sunset this evening Barry and I slog through a foot of snow walking the dogs around the cornfield. They leap and bound through the white like puppies and I trudge behind getting sweaty and feeling wonderful in the crisp air. A few clouds lie along the horizon and when the sun settles itself into the spires of the distant pines, the clouds turn all colors of pale pink, lavender and gray while the huge arch of sky above us becomes delicate blue. The landscape has taken on a magical aura. In the east a waxing moon brightens the darkening sky and off the tip of its crescent hangs a star, which reminds me while life may imitate art, it's really the other way around.

Back home at my desk, once again distracted from my writing, I gaze of out my window into the rapidly dimming dusk light. The doe has returned and this time she's brought her twins to dine at the feeder. I'm quite sure she's the one I saw crossing the street last spring when the twins were very small. I'm riveted to the window until the three have had their fill and melt into the brush.

On this eve of the New Year I think back over the past months and know that I've been given something special; I know that connecting with all the creatures who inhabit my neighborhood and all of the earth will forever nurture my soul. The flowers, the weeds, the dragonflies, butterflies and beetles; the elephants, the lions and white-tailed deer; the titmice, sparrows, chickadees and even the crows will dance in my imagination. And though I may not have named my love, may not yet call it faith, without question I know that nature sustains me with her constant wisdom and guidance and I know that belonging to my community of friends nourishes my soul. The practice of living moment by moment as best I know how has opened up a whole new world. It's allowed me to glimpse what has been there in front of me all the time. For this I feel a deep sense of gratitude. I may never be "cured" of what ails me, but I'm being healed by seeing myself as a whole being, by understanding how I fit into nature's scheme and finally, by coming to terms with my mortality a little at a time. I know death is part of the life I've been given. I mustn't live haphazardly but with intention, so I may be experiencing every moment I'm alive.

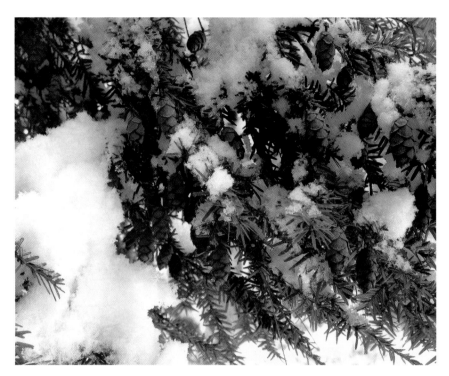

## *The Snow Storm*

I thought it was the promise
of white drifts that lured us into the dark,
into the stillness of falling snow.

Our fingers thread together.
You blow hard on mine
then lick a flake off my lip.

The hemlock shrugs its mantle of snow.
We collapse into its softness and flail
our arms into angel wings.
When we rise to behold the blackest west
a wind too high to feel has scoured the sky.

So tell me.
What drew us from the crackling fire, the ochre lamplight?
Have I imagined this unimaginable breath
that's blown a storm away and exhaled stars
like confetti across the sky so bright I can see your face?

# A Question of God

On and off for most of my life I've wondered about God—not with any particular urgency, but with an enduring curiosity, which nudged my imagination and hung around in the background of my thoughts. Recently this curiosity has elbowed its way to the forefront of my thinking and ripened into a desire to see if there's such a thing as a faith that might sustain me when all else fails. I've been suspicious of the word "faith." In an institutional religious context faith suggests to me absolutism, chauvinism, arrogance, bigotry and political exclusivity. The word brims not with glory, but with the messier aspects of human nature disguised by adherence to a particular faith.

I've been confused by religious traditions, theologies and churches, which claim theirs is the one true God and lay claim to the one and only truth. Religious institutions once ignored the Holocaust and we still wage holy wars in the name of God. I'm neither a true cynic, nor an atheist and I certainly don't begrudge anyone their personal faith so long as it isn't harmful to others or forced on me. I haven't been sure who God is or if one even existed. Intellectually I've conceded there's a powerful spirit in the universe, which is grander, by far, than anything I have experienced or can conceive of. This I know. Until recently this knowledge hadn't penetrated deep in my bones.

When I was a child, God wasn't in my family's vocabulary except on holidays, as a minor expletive or a bedtime ritual when I was told to pray that the Lord would keep my soul if I should die in my sleep. God was mentioned at Christmas when my mother read us *The Littlest Angel* and *Amahl and the Night Visitors* and these stories were no more than lovely fairy tales to me. Santa Claus and the Easter bunny took precedence over God on religious holidays until one winter when I was eight years old and my mother decided God was missing in her daughters' lives. (I hadn't been aware He figured much in hers.) She decided my sister and I should attend church.

Our erratic religious education began that winter. Agoraphobic and too anxious to leave the safety of her home, my mother prevailed upon our stepfather to escort my sister and me to Sunday services at the local Unitarian Church in Concord. She outfitted us in special holiday garb; matching fur-trimmed gray tweed hats, coats and leggings. I detested being dressed like my sister so I was off to a less than auspicious introduction to religion. Each Sunday my stepfather pulled on his old brown tweed coat and donned his tattered felt fedora with an audible sigh of resignation and graciously escorted us to the big white church in town. He'd taken precious time out from his farm chores to accommodate his new wife's whim—a mission to provide her daughters a proper religious education.

The Unitarian Church was a plain, wooden structure built in the simple, elegant style of many New England churches. It was topped with a tall white steeple housing a huge, white-faced clock whose golden hands wound around the hour until a sonorous bell tolled the time—the knell reverberated over the town. Inside the church cushionless hardwood pews rejected our bony backsides, and worn blue hymnals hung in racks on the back of the pew in front of us. Everywhere I looked the view was plain and unadorned until I'd lift my eyes to the tall, clear-paned windows and see the perfect blue of the winter sky, or the glittery green of a maple's new spring leaves, or the sunny yellow of its fall regalia. Except on those occasions when farm emergencies took precedence, my sister and I sat obediently in our pew beside our stepfather. When the hay had to be brought in before it rained, when a cow needed help calving or when the snow was too deep for travel I gloried in the freedom of those Sunday mornings.

My sister and I valiantly labored to pay attention to the minister's long-winded sermon stifling yawns behind our fists. We weren't allowed to squirm and this was particularly difficult under the circumstances. I remember how the minister's monotonous voice faded into the background of my reverie as I gazed out of the windows at the sky. It felt as if I were under water, just barely able to hear the distant voice far above me. Frequently, I was elbowed awake when my head dropped on my chest, but when it was time to sing a hymn, my stepfather's enthusiastic off-key rendition of "Onward Christian Soldiers" never failed to grab our attention and send my sister and me into uncontrollable giggles.

In the end it was the music that stirred me. My heart swelled with each crescendo raining down on us from the huge brass pipe organ in the loft at the back of the church. Listening to the rich soprano voice of the choir soloist convinced me that even if I couldn't see "God our Father," at least I could hear an angel. Forbidden to turn around to see what this angel looked like, it was left to my imagination to conjure up a lovely beatific-faced angel with soft white wings folded on her back. Looking down into my pew she sang just for me and when the organ changed key and the choir joined the heavenly soloist in her refrain, I was filled to bursting. I too, sang loudly with all my heart in my thin, passionate soprano voice until the hymn ended and the spell was broken.

The collection box affixed to the end of a long stick was passed down each pew and I had to give up the precious quarter my mother had seeded my pocket with, a quarter, which would have bought me quite a lot at the Five and Ten. The minister asked his congregation to kneel and pray to "our Father who art in heaven." As a child I was puzzled by having to pray to my father who really lived down south, not in heaven. Heaven was a place from which you never returned. How could the father I prayed to forgive my trespasses when he wasn't ever there to catch me trespassing—which was sneaking through a neighbor's yard, which I did a lot—unless my mother tattled on me, which I didn't think she would. The rest of the prayer eluded me completely, but I memorized it because I was told to do so, just as I did the prayer my mother had me say when she tucked me into bed at night. "Now I lay me down to sleep. I pray the Lord my soul to keep." I learned it for her and for the time she spent with me alone. "If I should die before I wake, I pray the Lord my soul to take." What did that mean? Might I die in my sleep? And why did the Lord want my soul? My unrelenting questions finally taxed my mother's patience to the limit and when she no longer was able to come up with creative answers, she'd tell me, "That's just the way it is, Holly" or "because I say so." I felt defeated and unsatisfied by these lame answers to burning questions, which prickled my small soul questions about life and death (and later, sex) and stopped asking. I never said this prayer with my own children when I said good night to them years later. Even then I hadn't any plausible explanation for what a soul was.

It wasn't long before Sunday attendance at the Unitarian Church dwindled down to a couple of times a month and finally to staying home. I don't think our churchgoing lasted more than a year. Perhaps my mother relinquished her fervent commitment to have someone else teach us about God, but more likely, my stepfather had become weary of wasting his time with two children who couldn't have been less interested in church. And not being a churchgoer himself I suspect he let my mother know he had better things to do with his time.

As the years passed and I grew older I occasionally attended the church services of different denominations as if sampling each to find the right one for me. None fit. None caught my imagination or touched my spirit. In fact, most of the services felt stodgy and confining. They seemed more about deferring to fallible human intermediaries who claimed expertise in matters concerning God and who didn't suffer questions and doubts any better than did my mother when I was a curious child.

Most puzzling was the notion of a loving God who judged my every thought, feeling and behavior and who had the power to punish me for any one of them just as my parents did when they chose to use or abuse this authority. I was also confused by a God who would erase my sins if I said, "I'm sorry" enough. I was frequently forced to apologize at home and was still not absolved of my misdeeds. I dismissed the notion of God's forgiveness.

In spite of all my youthful questioning and rejection of yet another father figure in my life, I never stopped loving the music or the sacred context in which it resounded. My spirit still soars with angels whenever I hear a choir sing. I once thought if God existed, it was because when I entered a cathedral I sensed something magical when the sun flung gleaming rainbows through stained glass windows into the silence. I've yet to put my finger on what it is that makes this magic. I wonder if it comes from the spirits of the cathedral builders, the carpenters of plain white churches who still linger in the palpable stillness of their monuments to God. Or maybe it's being part of a community in prayer that I can sense a power I can't name. Or maybe it's when I suddenly find myself catching my breath listening to the harmony of voices singing a hymn of hope. I know my soul is touched when tears spring unbidden to my eyes as I strain to reach the notes of the "Hallelujah"chorus—my passion exceeding my vocal ability. All of this celebrates the human spirit and it all reverberates through a community gathered to honor what is best in each of us. Those who built with spirit in their hands and hearts, the voices, which sing of that spirit, are truly felt in places of worship. Nevertheless, my long-held skepticism about the existence and efficacy of God ruled. Now and again questions did bubble up out of the dark and more often than not they quickly ebbed back where they came from.

When I was clubbed over the head with a life-threatening diagnosis, my expectable world capsized and once again questions deluged me. Unlike the profound questions that tumbled out of my youthful innocence, I was filled with an unstoppable urgency to find meaning and value in my life as I confronted the possibility of my own death. I was desperate for answers to fundamental mysteries, like why does a loving, all-knowing, powerful God blink when terrible things happen to people—not just disease, but Holocausts, wars in God's name and the general meanness that infects the messy world of humans? Was the God I'd learned about oblivious to the evil destroying the world he created? Where in the nature of things does badness come from? More and more I've come to realize, it's not God's job to mediate our human fiascos. It's our responsibility to deal with the pain, meanness and death that are part of being alive and human, that along with all creatures we're subject to the hard side of life.

If we're the only animal aware of our mortality and if we're the only animal who wishes to transcend this life, to find meaning in it, are we blessed or cursed by this intelligence? We abuse ourselves and each other and our environment when we have the capacity to choose to do otherwise. How come? Is it possible we're hard-wired to be both selfish for the sake of survival as well as to be communal, loving beings?

Confounded by what I'd found to be the narrow belief systems and chauvinism of many Christian churches, I've been looking for a believable, consistent and compassionate voice to help me find the answers I'm searching for or to understand there may not be any. I've read enough psychology to know how its concepts fit into my schema of the world. I've delved into books on spirituality, religion, nature and natural history and quantum physics. Undaunted by the enormous choice in the bookstores, I scanned the titles of unfamiliar authors, and particular books seemed to jump out at me just when I was ready to absorb their contents. This phenomenon continues now as I persevere in my spiritual exploration. So while I haven't made an exhaustive study of religion or of spirituality, I think I've learned enough to get a feel for where the journey is taking me and I've begun to piece together the rudiments of a spiritual philosophy that feels right.

I'm convinced the deep-seated anxiety I've experienced since getting cancer isn't neurotic; instead, it stems from the underlying fear that attends the thought of my own extinction. I wonder if this isn't why I need to give meaning and value to the pain and suffering that is part of my living, as well as to my inexorable journey toward death. I've learned there are pervasive and ancient thoughts in the world, which seem to have come from a universal soul or intelligence. Judaic, Buddhist, Christian, Islamic and Native American traditions share much in common. Indeed the voices of the prophets of the world's three major religions heard in the Talmud, the New Testament and the Koran appear to speak with the same universal language, which calls on us to attend to our innate drive to transcend ourselves, to think beyond ourselves, to love, to be kind, compassionate and forgiving and finally to understand that if we persist in searching we'll find God first within ourselves, then in the Universe.

Reading and pondering and walking in nature has led me to see there's a power or spirit residing in everything on earth: in rocks, deep in oceans, in trees and green things, in all creatures from elephants to dragonflies. It's the very same force of life that exists in me at a cellular level. Can it be that what I perceive as the potential for evil—the brutality of survival, natural disasters—is as much part of the universe as is the breathtaking beauty of the natural world and the potential for love? The notions of divine intelligence and intelligent design stir me, especially since I've just found out that my great, great grandfather, Louis Agassiz, believed in divine intelligence. I marvel at the infinitely complex universe in which I live and I'm particularly fascinated by the meticulously fashioned strands of DNA, which have determined what and who I am. I'm awed, as he must have been, by the extraordinary patterns in nature, the regularity of the seasons, the rising and setting of the sun and moon, the night sky filled with constellations, the birth, survival, and death of all creatures, and finally what appears to be both the randomness and the order of natural events. I can only wonder at Nature's elegant, infinitely complex and sacred design.

I don't wear a golden fur coat and I don't have wings or fins, but I share this force of life, this design with all living creatures. Like the dragonfly and the heron I survive as best as I can, but what I'm exquisitely conscious of, that they may not be, is that my life is finite. No matter how much I occasionally wish to stop time, no matter how much I yearn for balance and stability, I'm forced to accept change as inevitable.

Thinking about change, I realize that in my life changes have happened as a result of deliberate as well as unconscious choices with a bit of serendipity thrown in for good measure. I'm blessed and bedeviled by the fact I have some capacity to determine my destiny with the elements of good and bad residing in me. I've needed to overcome what makes me squirm inside about myself, to either overcome my frailties or learn to be more accepting of the parts of me I don't like and cultivate those that I do. I scuffle with choices daily, but my biggest struggle is letting go of the illusion of control—a most difficult hurdle for me. The Buddha says, "Everything that has a beginning has an ending. Make your peace with that and all will be well." It's hard for me to make peace with the knowledge of my eventual extinction. I find all my thoughts about spirituality, my spirit, and indeed, who I am, collide in the ultimate question—what will it be like not to be? In the process of coming to an understanding, I still have a long way to travel, but I'm trying to make the trip with a touch of grace and equanimity.

In the end, I've learned that whenever I still myself long enough to go within, to uncover my soul, I get closer to a place of acceptance and perhaps even faith. I trust persistent seeking will bring me even closer to what is best in me—love.

Wrestling with the question of God has, if nothing else, allowed me to know that getting breast cancer wasn't my fault or God's, it just happened. Was it a random occurrence? Was it something in the environment, did it happen for a purpose? Who knows? I can intervene to assist in my own healing, but my healing—or not—is part of the relationship I have with Nature and the nature within me over which I have little control—a humbling fact whenever I'm consumed with fear of recurrence. For now I can accept what I'm learning, at least intellectually, because it really does make sense to me, but the thinking is difficult, tricky, albeit compelling and much of the work I must do alone. One needs courage to delve into the dark places of one's soul.

I believe much of what I'm looking for is already inside me, that the seeds of healing have lain dormant in my soul. I believe in the power that brings me the gift of life, but I want to hear the joyful voice within sing louder than the voice that croons seductively from the dark corners of doubt.

I need to remind myself that a better day will, without doubt, follow a hopelessly gloomy one. I need to love and be nourished by the loving company of friends and family. I need to cherish solitude and walk daily into Nature to sustain peace inside myself. I need to listen carefully to the song of the homely brown sparrow and to breathe deeply. Although none of my thoughts about spirit and soul are set in stone, my life is starting to make more sense and feels more tolerable. And as I continue this journey into a spiritual place, I may not yet have faith in the theological sense, but I'm open to it, and I'm open to becoming more real by taking the risk of being more vulnerable. I feel like I'm unbuttoning my shirt to reveal my disfigured breast and still loving my body, because it's the one I have. It's a beginning.

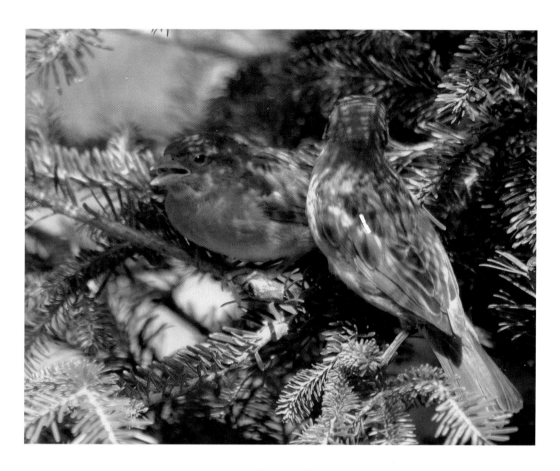

## A New Year

This much I know;
I wear my face
in dappled light with less regret.
I've taken root
like an old elm tree; I lean against north winds
rocking my house,
content to dance in place
knowing music
comes from inside out.
Where else shall I go to find
what I already know?
How else shall I be surprised?

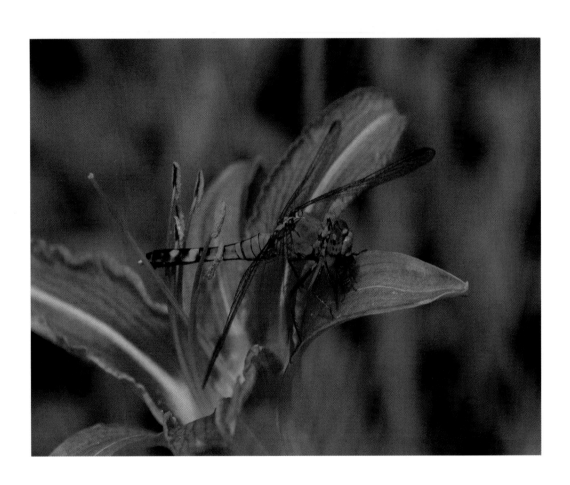

# Dancing With the Dragonfly II

I've heard the dragonfly say, dance
before she flashed her wings
and spun out of sight
across the ebony pond.

Again and over again,
I'll rise
to dance with her
in dreams, in daylight, at dusk.

If I tire,
if I forget or become dispirited,
the dragonfly will find me;
I'll breathe the air I'm in,
I'll quicken to bite a dappled pear.
I'll sing with a dolphin and dance with the wind .
I'll remember the feel of an elephant's hide,
the tiniest kiss on my nose.
I'll remember how petals fall like stars
to light my somber landscape.
Again and over again
I'll dance with the dragonfly
across
the ebony pond.

# GOOD READING

Armstrong, Karen. *A History of God.* New York: First Ballantine Books Edition, 1994.

Brown, Lauren. *Grasses, An Identification Guide.* New York: Houghton Mifflin, 1979.

Capra, Fritjof. *The Tao of Physics.* Boston: Shambhala Publications, 2000.

Carson, Rachel. *Silent Spring.* Boston: Houghton Mifflin, 1962.

Epstein, Mark. *Thoughts Without a Thinker.* New York: Basic Books, 1995.

———. *Going to Pieces Without Falling Apart.* New York: Broadway Books, 1999.

Fowler, George. *Learning to Dance Inside.* Orlando: Harvest Book, 1996.

Fox, Matthew and Rupert Sheldrake. *Natural Grace.* New York: First Image Books, 1997.

Frankl, Viktor. *Man's Search for Meaning.* New York: Pocketbook Editions, Washington Square Press, 1977.

Gibran, Kahlil. *The Prophet.* New York: Walker and Co., 1923.

Goodenough, Ursula. *The Sacred Depths of Nature.* New York: Oxford University Press, 1998.

Gray, Elizabeth Dodson. *Sacred Dimensions of Women's Experience.* Wellesley, Massachusetts: Round Table Press, 1988.

Hopes, David Brendan. *A Sense of the Morning.* Minneapolis: Milkweed Editions, 1999.

Kabat-Zinn, Jon. *Wherever You Go, There You Are.* New York: Hyperion, 1994.

Lindbergh, Anne Morrow. *Gift From the Sea.* New York: Pantheon Books, 1983.

Lurie, Edward and Louis Agassiz. *A Life in Science.* Baltimore: Johns Hopkins University Press, 1988.

Martz, Sandra, ed. *When I Am an Old Woman I Shall Wear Purple.* Watsonville, California: Papier-Mache Press, 1987.

Murdock, Maureen. *The Heroine's Journey.* Boston: Shambhala Publications, 1990.

Nisker, Wes. *Buddha's Nature.* New York: Bantam Books, 1998.

Raymo, Chet. *Natural Prayers.* St. Paul, Minnesota: Hungry Mind Press, 1999.

Shepard, Odell, ed. *The Heart of Thoreau's Journals.* New York: Dover Publications, 1961.

Shinoda-Bolen, Jean. *Close to the Bone.* New York: Touchstone, 1998.

Thich Nhat Hanh. *The Miracle of Mindfulness.* Boston: Beacon Press, 1975.

———. *Living Buddha, Living Christ.* New York: Riverhead Books, 1995.

Thoreau, Henry David. *Walden.* New York: Signet Classic, New American Library, 1999.

Tully, Mark. *Four Faces.* Berkeley: Ulysses Press, 1997.

Valentine, J. O., ed. Thoreau: On Land. New York: Houghton Mifflin, 2001.

Wilson, Edward O. *In Search of Nature.* Washington, D.C.: Island Press, 1996.

Wright, Mabel Osgood, ed., and Daniel J. Phillippon. *The Friendship with Nature.* Baltimore: Johns Hopkins University Press, 1999.

# Give the Gift of

## *Learning* to *Dance* With the *Dragonfly*

## to Your Friends and Colleagues

CHECK YOUR LEADING BOOKSTORE OR ORDER HERE

❑ **YES**, I want _____ copies of *Learning to Dance With the Dragonfly* at $29.95 each, plus $4.95 shipping per book (Massachusetts residents please add $1.50 sales tax per book). Canadian orders must be accompanied by a postal money order in U.S. funds. Allow 15 days for delivery.

My check or money order for $_____ is enclosed.

Name _____

Organization _____

Address _____

City/State/Zip _____

Phone_____ E-mail _____

*Please make your check payable and return to:*

### DANCING DRAGONFLY PRESS
867 Curve Street
Carlisle, MA 01741

*Or order at* **www.dancingdragonflypress.com**